For my lover, my best friend, my tall beautiful dark man!

from the
TABOO CONVERSATIONS
series

THAT SEX BOOK

HOW TO TALK ABOUT AND GET A HOT SEX LIFE AFTER 50

Dixie Maria Carlton

Contents

Behind Closed Doors ...   1

Chapter 1: Enjoying Great Sex After 50   5
Chapter 2: Who's Still Doing It and Why Does It Matter?   13
Chapter 3: From the Kama Sutra to Shades of Grey   23
Chapter 4: The Beauties and the Beasts   29
Chapter 5: How to Attract a Great Mate!   37
Chapter 6: Dating is Darned Hard Work After 50   43
Chapter 7: Getting Caught With Your Pants Down   51
Chapter 8: Princesses with Tarnished Tiaras   59
Chapter 9: Do We Grow Out of Slutty Behavior, or Into it?   67
Chapter 10: The Death of a Delicious Dream   73
Chapter 11: Condoms, Contraception, and Hair   79
Chapter 12: Now, Let's Get into the Good Stuff ...   89
Chapter 13: Seduction Is Not Just About the Sex   95
Chapter 14: The Golden Age of Intimacy   101

Chapter 15: Anticipation is a Powerful Aphrodisiac!   107

Chapter 16: Playtime – Getting Down to It   113

Chapter 17: Let's Talk About Toys   121

Chapter 18: You Show Me Yours – First!   131

Chapter 19: Having to Schedule Sex   139

Chapter 20: Spontaneity Derailment   145

Chapter 21: Slow Sex, Secret Sex, or No Sex at All   151

Chapter 22: What Boys and Girls Really Talk About ...   157

Chapter 23: The Orgasm Is No Longer the Objective   165

It's Not About the Sex!   171

Sex Trivia – or Did You Know ...   179

About Dixie Carlton   183

Acknowledgements   185

Sex past the age of 90
is possible – proving that
age does not matter.

Behind Closed Doors ...

Have you ever driven down a street of houses and wondered what's going on inside each one? Or looked up at an apartment block and considered the reality of the lives going on there? People are loving, fighting, struggling for survival, hooked on soap operas, eating peanut butter sandwiches for dinner, paying bills, crying on the bathroom floor, preparing to meet their partner's new family, masturbating, freaking out, watching you drive by ... No one knows what's going on inside, except those who are there, and maybe a best friend or two. When we get to 50, we're already well experienced in many of these things, and then life takes on a few new challenges doesn't it.

For many of us, we may wonder if it might be easier to be lonely and single vs lonely inside a bad relationship – and we weigh these things up carefully don't we. Those of us willing to take a chance on finding a new love, or returning to the deepest questions about rejuvenating our current relationship are the men and women I've written this book for.

And Sex – yes, we need to talk about Sex. Because sex is one of the most important things for so many of us. Even more than in our teenage years, our mid/post-midlife bodies are hormonal, hungry, and no one seems to believe us that yes, sexuality and sensuality are still mightily important later in life. And what's the new normal? Is there one? How do we navigate the rocky terrain of getting what we want in the bedroom and what we need to compromise on? Because we're so much better at that now too, right?

So, let's have a friendly chat about all these things. Some of what you may be curious about – or be asking Google for more information about before you talk to your best friends – is likely to be covered here. But the main message I want to drive home, is that talking about all these things could mean make a huge difference to your ability to maximize your horizontal happiness.

So, let's (change how we) talk about sex ... baby!

Sexual pleasure is the legitimate right of every human being.

– *Samual Ann Wear*

Dancing is a perpendicular expression of a horizontal desire.

– George Berhard Shaw

CHAPTER 1

Enjoying Great Sex After 50

Where do I start?

This book was inspired by a conversation I had recently in a saucy little boutique near where I live. It's run by a lady I'll call Louise. I'd been there a few weeks earlier and bought a stunning little cotton dress that showed off my great legs and enhanced my newly re-discovered curves.

We joked about how the recent departure of my husband meant I'd lost 220lb of 'deadweight', and had also lost a few pounds myself. Yes! One small advantage of the stress of a marriage breakup means you stop eating properly and the weight you tried to shed during the "happy" years just falls away of its own accord.

For me, the end of my short-lived marriage just made me want to curl up and die for a while. I didn't see it coming and the feeling of failure was devastating. Then reality took over and I found that what I really wanted was to just get busy with getting on with my life and that meant re-evaluating a number of things.

When I first tried on that little white dress in Louise's shop, we joked about how it looked so great on me that I might even "get lucky". As it happened, I did wear that dress a few days later, and by chance I not only got lucky but got to know someone whom I very quickly grew to love and appreciate for so many things he has brought into my life. Soon I was back with Louise and telling her, "I'm so lucky that I'm now having the all-time best sex of my entire life". And I have to say – that was already a pretty high benchmark!

Louise remembered me from my earlier visit and introduced me to a friend of hers, Tammy, who happened to be there. It was a quiet day in the store, and before I knew it, I was enjoying a hot cup of tea with them and sharing some fascinating and intimate girl talk.

Tammy, it turned out, was in her mid-70s, and had been with her much younger lover for just on seven years. "Great sex is absolutely worth having," she declared. "And we all need more of it."

"That's true," said Louise – but she could barely remember the last time she had had *great* sex.

She did recall that sometimes great sex comes with moments of great confusion and recounted a time when the man she was with was delicious on all fronts – especially when on his hands and knees – but that he had no capacity for spontaneity. Realising that he was stopping to fold his undies as he took them off was a bit of a passion killer.

Tammy then advised that for a seriously good bonk, "it's often still a matter of having to rely on a dildo. At least that usually meant a measure of reliability, it's mess free, and seriously, who really needs a cuddle after!" All three of us roared with laughter.

This was not a conversation I expected to have with two strangers in their 60s and 70s respectively. But it was such fun!

Time flew by that day; new boots were purchased and friendships established. I will definitely be going back to Louise's for more hospitality, even if the conversation is not always quite so risqué!

Which brings me to my next point. The day before that little shopping trip, I found myself at the local drugstore asking for a morning-after pill. At 52, I had been so busy having so much fun that my hormones were suddenly all over the place. Though my periods had stopped nearly a year earlier, my body was suddenly starting to behave like I was 35 again. So, this was a precaution – if possibly an over-thinking, paranoid one – but hey, after being married for a while to someone who'd had a vasectomy, having to think about contraception again was a big oops moment.

Well-meaning friends were already advising me that STDs in the over-50s are very much on the rise. Because it took a while for me and my new man to actually get to dance the full horizontal mambo, the issue didn't really need addressing for a few weeks. But I can tell you it feels pretty darned weird to be standing before a 30-something, cute-as-a-button red-headed pharmacist asking for a Morning After Pill.

Cue the eyeroll. "The darned unpredictability of meno-pause" floats out of my mouth as she smiles and completes the sale. Maybe because she's a redhead like me, it was ok. She got it. Gals like us, according to various old wives' tales, are supposed to have the highest libidos.

At this point in history we are watching great TV shows like *Frankie and Grace*, with Jane Fonda starring as a corporate wannabe in the business of marketing vibrators to the 70-plus crowd. There are movies like *The Book Club* featuring more women over 70 having sex and getting hot and horny over the *50 Shades of Grey* series. But who's really writing about those of us in the thick of it, dating, and having outstanding sex, in our 50s and 60s?

Me.

That's who.

And what makes me an expert on this? I'm not a former sex worker, or a qualified sex therapist. In fact, I'm probably a lot more like you – the person reading this book. I'm someone from the suburbs who still looks like washed-up flotsam when I go to the gym and then straight to the supermarket. A regular woman who is not too tall, not too short, wears make up, gets her hair cut and styled every few weeks, stays in most nights and loves to cook. I might be overlooked in a city bar if out for a night with friends, but maybe might still attract a conservative onceover from the quiet guy at the cafe.

I've tried online dating – both successfully and unsuccess-fully – I've been married a couple of times, and I've slept with more men than some of my friends and a lot less than others.

But I like sex. I love the nuances, the mystery, the intrigue, and the intimacy of quality sex and lovemaking. I love to know how it works – how women and men make that magic happen. And so, I've been doing my best to casually study this since I was a teenager. Now, having decided to write this book about getting out and getting it at this age and stage of life, I'm exploring the subject further. I'm having even more exciting conversations about sex, menopause, men, dating, and horizontal fun in general. Yay!

Sex is always about emotions.
Good sex is about free emotions,
bad sex is about blocked emotions.

– Deepak Chopra

CHAPTER 2

Who's Still Doing It and Why Does It Matter?

I think we'd all be surprised to know that having sex in old age is not only possible, but very enjoyable. As I was researching stories for this book I learned about a couple in their 80s who enjoyed a jaunt into their local high-quality lingerie and adult toy store. They bought up large, saying they "really wanted to experiment some more."

But before we go there, let's look at what we are told by our friends. Just as we did in our in our puberty years, we talk amongst ourselves and form conclusions based on what our best friends are doing and saying – and on what we read in *Cosmopolitan*, *O Magazine* and online. Fortunately for all of us, *Sex and the City* brought sex right out into the open between 1998 to 2004 and made it okay for us to delve deeper. Girlie chats became more open. Then *50 Shades of*

Grey allowed us to share some of what gets us hot, or not, and the truth about who was still "doing it" over 40 was out.

Most of us were, but many of us were not having a lot of fun with it.

Our men were inept or, in many cases, were told fibs too often by frustrated or bored women who kept saying, "Yes, baby, that was great" and "No, I did not fake my orgasm". Sadly, that has led to far too many men believing they are far better at sex than they really are. After years of only hearing applause, a man is quite bewildered if he receives any negative feedback. That's when we're asked, "What's wrong with you?" Or, "Why can't you women all play the same game?" No wonder men are confused.

Those of us who did fake it have done so with little compassion for the women who would follow in our footsteps. Is footsteps the right word? Well, you know who you are, and yes, we've all been guilty of it at some time or another.

Some of us simply don't care and are used to just lying back like starfish and letting it happen. Others have never actually experienced good sex anyway, and so have no idea what all the fuss is about. Those in that category happily shut up shop early and hang up their libidos like the size-too-small jeans they wore back in the day. Maybe some keep their urges hidden in a drawer somewhere to bring out just in case the chance ever comes around again, but often the "use it or lose it" rule becomes a reality.

Some men also decide at various ages that they don't want to endure an ongoing sex life either and just as happily zip up their flies so their dicks are then used purely for peeing out of. Perhaps they do this to avoid addressing their perceived issues of malfunction or inadequacy. And maybe women give up due to dryness, or issues with contraception or just because good sex is so hard to find.

I was at a women's group evening recently where an attractive woman of 58 said she'd recently been hit on and had no idea why. After all, she felt she was "no longer a sexual being". When pressed, she said she did not take up the offer and laughed it off. I wanted to ask more, as I was curious about why she felt that way.

Unfortunately, there's a frequent mismatch between those who want to play and those who don't.

Some people say they can tell if a woman is still having sex. There's a certain jauntiness, or twinkle in her eye. She may still dress to attract and has an undercurrent of flirty about her. That's not to say she is *actually* having sex, especially if she's single, but there are those who are open to the possibility and those who aren't. I believe we can often recognize those we can have "those conversations" with versus those who will quickly change the subject.

My hairdresser expressed this thought eloquently when she said, "We can always tell who's getting it and who's not. Even their hair bounces better!"

In this age of equality, and openness, why can't we talk more about it? Who's to say we can't learn a lot from each other? Perhaps that's where we are best to focus our attention. If we're reasonably certain the friends we talk with are still having great sex, why not talk about what we do, how much fun we have, and even what new and interesting things we may have learned as we got older.

I first developed a fascination for sex when I was a horny teenager, assisted by my then boyfriend. Access to his *Penthouse* magazine collection meant I could devour insights from Xaveria Hollander. She was a famous former call girl who wrote a best-selling book called *The Happy Hooker: My Own Story.* At 16, I read her advice on how to do, er ... "some things" and studied her articles far more intently than anything my English teacher assigned us to read.

While some of my friends were discovering smoking, drinking, Pat Benatar and weed, I was making the most of the fact that in the early 1980s, the worst thing that might happen was pregnancy. As long as you were on the Pill and you were careful about your reputation, you could study sex without any serious consequences.

And so, I did.

I also read everything I could get my hands on, including *The Joy of Sex* and the *Kama Sutra,* and was lucky enough to have a boyfriend who was also curious and willing to learn.

That's not to say I didn't have sex droughts, or bad sex over the years, but I always liked to learn about it and took pride in being reasonably good at it. Perhaps this is due to my being a natural redhead. As already noted, some research says it's my apparent instinct to really like sex. Redhead or not, I like consensual, wholesome, mutually satisfying sex. And what's not to like? Really!

The arrival of Aids and increased awareness of other STDs in the 1980s did slow most of my generation down a bit, but for many of us sex was something to be enjoyed. While our mothers and grandmothers had to keep pretty darned quiet about it, my generation was allowed to be a *little* more open and honest about sex.

Adult stores, toys, and even sex expos became a lot more open to ordinary folks outside the porn business in the 1990s. For those of us in our 30s and 40s, the sexual revolution was taking a few giant steps forward. We saw the first lesbian kisses on TV, sex became increasingly mainstream as a subject and was even shown quite blatantly on some shows. It all started to change our thinking about sex and we ramped up our conversations accordingly. *Sex and the City* helped us open up so much more and, two decades later, we can look back and appreciate just how far we've come. No pun intended!

What Are We Doing – Really?

Those of us who have fun with sex usually started out that way because, first and foremost, it has always been fun. It is safer fun than drugs or alcohol, even if still not recommended while driving a car or operating machinery! We are by and large conditioned to a certain level of "normal" but with a side of "kinky". Isn't it funny how even the kinky word is no longer kinky?

So, what *is* the new normal?

On top, straight sex, blow jobs, oral sex, dildos, vibrators, sex outdoors, threesomes, anal sex, gay sex, exploring bi-sexuality – all these terms are classified as being within the range of normal by most people I know who are still having good or great sex over 50. Maybe not *all* these things are, but about 70 per cent of these concepts are terms we're all intimately familiar with. Or at the very least have tried, or come close to trying.

I once went to a sex party, that was like a Tupperware party. The woman hosting it was a friend and the presenter was someone I also knew, although not well. She talked about all the devices and toys she had brought with her to sell and shared how she had taken her job so seriously that she had "hung out with a dominatrix". She'd wanted to research everything that was on the table that night and so had learned first-hand about S & M, domination, pain as a stimulant, and much more.

I am personally not interested in this side of life, and most of my friends and those I've had a gazillion conversations with are not either, so I'm not going to go into too much detail here. A good smack on the bum at the right moment is about as far as I'd personally go in the pain department. But the interesting thing is, we are all more aware of such preferences now – especially since *50 Shades of Grey* arrived as a runaway bestseller in 2011. Whether or not we are personally into any particular "thing", we are at least willing to talk about it. Maybe even speculate a little.

Fetishes are also more commonly talked about and understood. Having someone lick your toes, brush your hair, rub your feet, dress up in particular costumes, feed you certain things while tied up or enjoy a whole host of "slight" oddities is one thing. The extremes of fetishism can open up some dark and strange places.

What is normal for one, however, is maybe too out there for someone else. But let's not judge each other for our personal desires. So long as no one is being hurt or totally freaked out, let's say, for the sake of this book, that normal consensual sex is whatever we personally want it to be.

Everything that makes us happy is quite simple. Love, sex, food.

-Meryl Streep

CHAPTER 3

From the Kama Sutra to Shades of Grey

I remember, years ago, finding out there was an ancient book called the *Kama Sutra*. All I knew was that it was about all the many sexual positions that lovers enjoy and everyone wanted to get their hands on a copy. When E. L James's *50 Shades of Grey* series came along, it had everyone all aflutter too.

By the time the *Kama Sutra* had done its rounds, most people were clear that while there might technically be dozens of positions, there were really only a handful that were workable – even for those of us who might try being acrobatically inclined. Our own imaginations soon also helped us realize there was a lot more to good sex than how many positions you might know.

So, back to the question of "normal". Sure, one person's "normal" may be another person's "weird". But one thing is for sure: the older we get and the more experienced we become, the more we open up to ideas and options that might once have been considered taboo, both by us and society in general.

With maturity comes a willingness to take our time and explore a little. For many of us, the kids are likely to be grown up by the time we get to our 50s. By then, the urgent *need* for satisfaction often gives way to the desire for longer, more fulfilling sessions of lovemaking. The days of desperately wanting to get it on anywhere, and as quickly as possible, fade away once we're no longer anxious about being discovered by our parents, waking the baby, or having our kids walk in on us. A little leisurely time spent together is often an option, allowing us to explore a little more behind closed doors. This might be a matter of touching more, giving or receiving massage, tickling behind the knees or figuring out if having our toes or feet licked is really fun or just a gross idea.

Some ideas for exploring might include:
- Head or foot massage;
- Having your hair brushed;
- Caressing (with either fingers, lips, or tongue) your lover's shoulders, arms, buttocks, thighs, neck, armpits, ankles, feet;
- Just kissing for a very long time;
- Enjoying toe play – surprisingly this can be incredibly erotic, though you want to be sure your feet are clean and well pedicured;Playing dress ups – either role playing or with lingerie;

- Being tied up, blindfolded, having your senses teased;
- Moving sex out of the bedroom – or at least the foreplay part;
- Introducing toys, flavored lubricants;
- Reading porn together – if you've never tried this together, you might be surprised how much you enjoy sharing a good bedtime story.

The point is, there may be new erogenous zones you never ever knew you had until you take the time to explore slowly and sensuously with a deliberate focus on the journey, not the destination.

You don't have to be age
20 or size zero to be sexually
viable, or viable as a woman.

-Belinda Carlisle

CHAPTER 4

The Beauties and the Beasts

If you think your "good old days" are gone, just ask anyone who finds themselves in a new relationship just *how* good the sex can be. Ask, too, how important that is compared to the bedroom activity they had with their partner of the past twenty years. That is not to say you need to trade in your old spouse or lover to rejuvenate your love life, but you can certainly gain new perspectives on the power of great sex within your current relationship by talking to people who are busy exploring new ones.

Outstanding sex is definitely not the domain of teens and horny young lovers. I'd go so far as to say that youth and great physical pleasures are *wasted* on the young. That also includes technology. Many of us in our middle years are having a fantastic time with online texting, Skyping, and all kinds of long-distance phone sex. After all, we are often traveling a lot in our later years, even while wanting to hold onto good relationships.

The young may find it hard to believe, but love is just as intense, sex is just as extraordinary, and feelings are every bit as deep in maturity as in youth. Maybe more so. In fact, according to many I've talked with, the frailties of life and the swift passing of time make us more likely to value the feelings we have for friends and lovers in our later years. Somewhere in our 40s we reach that point of certainty that life is short and we need to play harder. Make it all count more.

But first things first: how do we meet people these days? When we were young there were chances to meet potential partners at parties, pubs and other people's weddings. Nowadays, you're more likely to meet someone special at a funeral than a 21st birthday party.

Online dating is the easiest way to meet anyone these days. Or is it? We really do need to make it count all the more, because time is ticking, right? So we go online, put our profiles up and wait. And wait. And what comes up? Mostly it's disappointment. Sad but true. I have lost count of the stories I've heard from friends and acquaintances over 40 who have had to contend with liars, cheaters and people with totally unrealistic expectations.

They include men in their 60s trying to pass themselves off as two decades younger, who are seeking women in their 30s. On their wish lists are big boobs, flowing hair, long legs and asses that J-Lo would be proud of. Preferably there'll be no children in the picture. I'm not sure about the last time you thought of this, but older men don't usually dress to disguise their real age, so pretending to be 45 is just dumb. Also, women in their 30s who use dating sites are often single parents with teenagers or younger children who are holding down jobs and don't have time to just look fabulous. The only exceptions will be gals with money who don't need to work. They have time to get weekly nail/hair/beauty treatments, do daily gym workouts and employ a nanny to take care of the kids so they can actually date those older guys with unrealistic expectations.

Okay, I'm being cynical here, and yet we all see those reality shows that show us the image I've just conjured up. There are also far too many women lying about their age and not being authentic. We all know it.

What if we just all decided to put our best foot forward, present ourselves in the best way possible, and hope for the best because we have faith that *not everyone* is out to screw us over ... despite the best efforts of scammers to undermine that faith.

Let's consider the other kind of seeker on the dating sites – the people who are just unaware that they are punching well above their weight. Again, sorry for the extreme cynicism, but having been "smiled at" by enough toothless, shaggy-haired losers who barely own footwear, let alone a decent shirt ... need I explain?

As I began to write this book, a friend commented that far too many women in the 45-plus age group are just seeking a soft landing with a rich guy. I called him on this and explained that just as many guys in this age bracket have similarly unethical or unrealistic ideals. And then I considered again the number of amazing relationships I'm aware of that have stemmed from great online connections. Some have led to lasting, happy marriages.

Soul mates are found online, in the supermarket, at the sidelines of the game on Saturdays, signing up for marathons, doing volunteer work and in a whole range of places. There is no easy answer as to where or how you might meet someone, but don't give up on trying to find someone who is special, genuine, and wants the same things as you do. Online sites might also be riddled with scammers, bad guys, and dangerous characters, but so too were (and still are) the clubs, pubs, and backyards of friends.

Very few people can divorce themselves from what they feel emotionally and sexually.

-Boy George

CHAPTER 5

How to Attract a Great Mate!

About 10 years ago, I was having a deep and meaningful conversation with one of my favorite guy friends – there were tears, and tissues involved. We were both going through some heartache and we sat on the phone and talked about how hard it is to find a great partner. He suggested an idea that I've always liked and have also used myself.

Grab a journal or a large piece of paper and some colored pens and go somewhere quiet. You need lots of colors! You're going to tune into your rainbows and create a great mate – on paper.

Start by listing key points under the heading of My Perfect Partner. You don't have to be neat or write a bullet-point list – just write! Some points might include things like:

Attractive / Has nice friends / Gets on with his mother / Wants or has kids / Nice to sleep with / Good looking / Dresses well ...

On you go by adding, for instance, tall, blond, dark, hairy, bald, Christian, Muslim, Hindu, spiritual, non-religious, fit, loves dogs, loves cats, works with people, a geek, introvert, extrovert, loves ethnic food, good cook, experimental, likes sex, adventurous ...

You get the general idea, right?

Then, in another section of the page, or on a separate page, create your non-negotiable list. This is the most important part of the exercise, for you are now identifying and specifying key points around which you won't lower your standards.

You might make a few exceptions, of course. For example, my best friend loves bald men, especially tradesmen. But – if Mr Perfect turns up with a head full of hair and has the right star sign (after two failed marriages with hairy Scorpios she wasn't about to look at one of those), might she give him a second look? Sure, if he fills the bill in all other respects.

She could, for instance, always talk him into shaving his head if that was really important to her, or even grow to love his hair as it is. But a point like "no snoring or sleep apnea" might be a non-negotiable.

For a man, it might be quite different. Shaved female underarms might be on the non-negotiable list for some, and not for others. It's all about *you*, baby! Make your list the way *you* want it to be. You never have to share it with anyone, but you do need to have your key points clear in your own mind.

This is called "putting it out to the universe" in your search for Mr/Ms Right – someone who truly *fits* with you.

This process might sound odd to you, maybe even a little too "woo woo", but if you've been looking for a while and nothing else has worked so far, what do you have to lose? Seriously, this works. I know it from so many people who have vouched for it, and yes, it has worked for me too. It is not backed by scientific evidence but there is power in thinking about, and committing to paper, the kind of partner you really do want *and* the things about him or her you just won't tolerate.

Note that if you find yourself struggling to match or step up to what's on your list, then you might consider this as a sign to invest in some personal development or make a few changes to your own looks or habits. For example, wanting someone with a healthy attitude or firm body means you need to have these attributes, too. Seems obvious doesn't it, but it's a matter of balancing what we want and what we have to offer.

As my good friend Sue Lester, The Mindset Coach, said to me: "This is a crucial point as we attract the partner at the level we're at, so if you're struggling to be on par with what you are asking for, alarm bells should ring. Get help from an appropriate coach or counselor to build your self-esteem and confidence, or gain financial, health or career skills, to bring yourself up to the level you desire."

The only person who can truly fill the hole inside you is you. Failing to attend to your own growth is why people will go through a whole series of disastrous relationships or online dates and keep on attracting the same flavor, just in a different wrapper.

The only common denominator in all your relationships is you.

*Sexuality poorly repressed
unsettles some families,
well repressed it unsettles
the whole world.*

-Gore Vidal

CHAPTER 6

Dating is Darned Hard Work After 50

Dating's not easy when you hit your middle years. By then we know how valuable sex, love, and friendships are, and our feelings around these things are therefore arguably more intense. Dating at 50-plus can be immensely frustrating, challenging, and in some instances downright dangerous for one's mental health.

The amount of second guessing that goes on in our minds is second only to that of a puppy who knows he's not supposed to try and play with the family cat but just really, really wants to. The impulses are rampant, but the wisdom argues fiercely with the compulsion to just dive in, even when you know you're risking a nasty scratch or snarl.

One of the biggest challenges is finding out that while you might be a perfect fit at first, some pretty big compromises may need to be made to *maintain* that fit. I used to hear the old saying, "When the honeymoon is over, what will it be like then?" As a young person I really did not know what that meant. Of course, when you're in love you think honeymoons will go on for years. However, the older and more experienced or cynical we become, the more we realize honeymoons are really just that lustful phase of getting to know each other and enjoying the intense voyage of discovery.

The list of things you might put up with in a new partner increases as you grow older. And once we start counting the negatives – or talking about them with our best friends – we may realize that we could seem a little shallow.

Some 50-plus friends I know will simply not entertain the idea of dating anyone with school-age children. Some may be even more wary about kids in specific age bands. At least one female friend of mine endured a bout of step-parenting that left her with a PTSD diagnosis and a robust aversion to teenage girls.

Several friends have been advised by their lawyers not to date anyone with considerably less money than they have. Others will be turned off by observing the level of passion a prospective partner might have for fitness, sports and hobbies.

That's fair enough. If your last serious relationship saw you becoming a fishing or golf widow every weekend, why wouldn't you avoid dating someone with similar tendencies?

Some people feel very strongly that sex *has* to be part of, or definitely *not* part of, what's on offer.

And then there's the matter of net worth. Some people – both men and women – may seek a partner who is a step up for them. They may have come out of a past relationship with significantly diminished resources and think that finding a wealthier man or woman will be the answer to their prayers.

Sure, it takes the financial heat right off to find someone who wants what you want and is willing to foot the bill. Women are increasingly targeted by men who have lost at least half of everything in a marriage split to former wives. Such men find themselves moving closer to retirement age without as many eggs in their baskets as they used to have, or thought they'd have, in their 50s and 60s.

There are also women who do quite well out of marriage breakups and know how relatively easy it can be to repeat the process of finding another man to milk. While this might be a highly controversial thing to say, it is happening in many social circles.

Quite simply, there are a lot of desperately lonely people out there who are single-minded about rebuilding their finances the fast and easy way. Learning how to "be all that you want me to be" just to gain access to another person's soul (and bank account) is callous, dirty work but, as with any other well-rewarded job, there's always someone willing to do it.

On the other side of all that are the losers who inspire songs of heartbreak and despair. They also inspire lawyers to urge the rest of us to have rock-solid investments, pre-nuptial agreements and trusts, and to attend seminars on how *not* to have your heart, trust, and assets exposed to vultures!

I've known several women who've appraised men they

were dating on the grounds of their work, cars and addresses, simply because they feared these new loves might not be equal with them in terms of financial stability.

If this seems shallow, let's look at it further. If you are a woman who has raised her own family, saved and kept your own home and is also starting over in midlife, you'll have questions when you go out on a dinner date. Is it appropriate to pay half the bill? Should you drive and meet the guy at the restaurant, or have him take you there? Do you want a say in where you'll eat? What if you have no idea about his level of income and he turns up wearing a faded shirt or frayed jacket and seems to order the cheapest thing on the menu? You are going to read everything about him from his clothing, behaviour and attitude to what he orders.

I went out twice with a man who drove a very classy Mercedes, wore a nice suit and took me to a really lovely place down on the waterfront. The first time was lovely. The second date was considerably different. He was very attentive on the phone during the 10 days between dates, but turned up the second time with a smudge on his shirt. The car was his "other car", he said. This one was a scruffy, dirty 12-year-old gray sedan that smelled bad. We went to a place that was pay-as-you-order bistro. It was made clear that I was to pay for this second meal, and that he expected a lot more than a kiss goodnight.

When I asked about the car he actually told me he only brought out the Mercedes to impress. Most of the time he drove the "regular" car. Then it turned out that payments on the Mercedes were taking just about every cent he had, but he thought it might turn out to be a good long-term investment if he kept the mileage way down.

I don't really care what a man drives, but the subterfuge was a total turn off.

Here a few dating tips that might help both men and women.

Yes, guys, open the door for her – and if she doesn't like it and objects to your being polite, walk away. Anyone objecting to being treated like a decent person deserves to be ignored. And ladies, you could also try opening the door for him if you reach it first. Just be gracious in your behaviors. Keep it that simple.

Men, don't order off the menu for her – she's perfectly capable of doing that for herself. But by all means give her some recommendations if you are already familiar with the place.

Compliments are always appreciated. If you're going on a first date or an extra special date, chances are you may both put some thought into your appearance. In some instances you'll perhaps agonise over your choice of dress, shirt, shoes, and still change your clothes 16 times before getting out the door ... only to race back inside and change again. When you are complimented sincerely, that ridiculously large pile of changed outfits hastily tossed back into the wardrobe leaves your mind and you can sigh with relief and finally relax a bit. And compliments for guys are also important.

You may need to take some of your social cues from your partner. Things such as what to wear in bed, who makes the bed, where to eat, who pays, who cooks or cleans up after dinner can all be talked about or clarified as time goes by. Hygiene matters, such as cleaning teeth on waking, or having showers together, or not, leaving socks or towels on the floor etc ... may seem really small, but might also be irritation triggers for your new partner. In that case, you need to know how to pick your moments and bring these up for discussion.

I personally can't stand it when someone messily drops their knife and fork on the plate when they've finished eating. That's just my thing and it grates my gears. Good table manners in general are important to me. But if I really (and I mean *really, really*) liked a man in *every* other way, I'd feel it was worth mentioning what was frustrating me or turning me off.

One man I know refuses to finish a meal with a woman on a date if she has to take a photo of the meal and share to social media before they eat. At the end of the day, remember we're all adults with tongues in our heads and the right to say what we do and don't find attractive or acceptable in those we are spending time with.

It's about communication – we need much more of it.

A woman of my age is not supposed to be attractive or sexually appealing ... I just get kinda tired of that.

– Kathleen Turner

CHAPTER 7

Getting Caught With Your Pants Down

Cheaters are common at any age. It's just that by the time we're in our 50s, we're hoping those who do this have gotten the urge to stray out of their systems. We hope they have found what they really wanted in the smorgasbord of life and made some firm decisions around commitment. But sadly, "once a cheater, always a cheater" is ultimately a truism that can't be ignored.

It's easy to imagine that we're smart enough in middle age to recognize the signs of a cheating lover or spouse. But how do we spot the cavalier prick or bitch who is just out for what they can get? There are plenty of them. As mentioned earlier, some people can put on a great show to win the deal but have no idea about follow-through. Authenticity is rare. So is integrity.

I've lost count of the friends who've talked about an

"amazing" person with whom they have a "real connection" – only to find that all was not as it seemed at the start.

Maybe we should ask for a reference or treat dating like we would if hiring a nanny or a new business manager. After all, haven't we the right to know as much as possible at the start of a relationship?

I have dated a lot over the last few decades, and sometimes it was successful and other times a total disaster. A man who had seemed so lovely to me many years ago, turned out to be someone dedicated to targeting vulnerable younger widows. He knew all the right things to say and do, and before I knew it, he'd moved in and taken over my life! And not in a good way.

Scammers abound, unfortunately, and the most successful are smooth, well-practiced at the art of romantic subterfuge. My own experience led me to create a firm rule with my closest friends: *all future relationship prospects had to pass the friend test.*

This has gone on to become a fairly standard analysis of the pros and cons of dating partners. We all do it now for each other, and I know some of those friends have introduced it to other friends,

This goes beyond just having a "girlie chat over a few wines". It is instead an almost clinical review of the proposed partnership. We all have to agree to take these feedback sessions and consider them soberly and thoroughly before committing to a serious relationship. If we don't, then how can we expect to receive anything but their harshest I-told-you-so reminders when or if commiserations become necessary later on.

The way we've ended our own previous relationships can say a lot about us. Our exes know how much kindness of spirit and generosity we showed when the split-up happened. They can be our greatest champions, or harshest critics.

The next person who walks into your life might want to know – before committing their hearts to a relationship – that you are a good person who plays fair, keeps your word and means what you say.

It might help them to learn what upsets you, what triggers are best avoided, and what kind of amazing friend, lover and supporter you might be with the right partner.

After all, by the time we're in our 50s, it's starting to sink in that we have fewer years left for traveling the scenic route towards true love and *Happy Ever After Land*. All the help we can get would be great. *Why not ask for references?*

Online dating sites allow you access to personality profiles and the answers to many questions posed by the site managers, so you have a *reasonable* idea of what you're getting yourself into. Of course, players and cheaters have these things well worked out too. Trusting, vulnerable, honest people really don't stand a chance against someone who is fully intent on defrauding others and playing a good game. All you can really do is keep your wits about you, look for the signs of good, bad, and everything in between, and commit to a relationship based on transparency and clear communication.

Our pasts will make us naturally inclined to over-think things at times. So long as we can talk about those potential sore spots we'll most likely be okay, but they are best discussed when you're still getting to know each other, not when you're already hooked and in deep.

I recently talked with a man who has been married to his wife for more than 25 years. He said to me that he and his wife are still sexually active and happily so, enjoying sex several times a month. Sometimes it's every day or more than once a day. At other times a week might go by, but then they are "like rabbits" again.

Interestingly, though he is now totally faithful to his wife, it was different many years ago. He didn't detail the frequency or nature of his infidelities but did say he was over 40 before he came to understand the value of having a committed relationship with his wife. They worked out that what they had was very special. They're now both in their 60s and he feels very strongly that he cannot imagine being sexually intimate with anyone else again. She is the centre of his universe, and that is that.

Can men fall in love all over again with (their same) women in the midlife years? Maybe. Some men, however, are so in love with their partners from the start that the very idea of being unfaithful is simply beyond comprehension for them. This is not what many women believe of course – but my research tells me that some men simply are not willing to ever risk their marriages. This includes men who may not be "getting any" at home, or who may not even be in love with their partners any more or who may be less than happy in their relationships for any number of reasons. End of story.

I hope that for many women reading this, it's reassuring to

know that many men can be trusted, despite what the various women's magazines and reality TV shows might suggest. A *lot* of men, and women, do have very high standards and stick to them.

The behaviour of a human being in sexual matters is often a prototype for the whole of his other modes or reactions in life.

– *Sigmund Freud:* Sexology and the Psychology of Love

CHAPTER 8

Princesses with Tarnished Tiaras

If you have already raised your own family and are enjoying some personal and financial freedom, why would you want to put your own retirement and lifestyle plans on hold to accommodate the unplanned arrival in your life of other people's children?

If you have raised sons you might find girls to be hard work, and their ways very foreign to that of boys. If you're used to girls around your home, you may struggle with your partner's boys or building a new family that combines both.

The way you parent might leave you open to thinking your partner's offspring get away with things you wouldn't permit. And woe betide anyone criticizing your own parenting style. Of course, we all think our own kids are better than everyone else's.

Finding a wonderful new partner in life after the age of 50

can be quite simply exhilarating, but not at the expense of all our hard-won lifestyle gains. Have we not earned the right to be a little bit selfish?

If after years of raising a family and the chance for happiness with a new partner comes along, is it selfish of us to want it? I've known some people who took years off from having a social life or dating in order to focus on their kids and then found it very hard to give themselves permission to focus on their own needs.

At some point our kids do grow up and leave, and we're left wondering if shedding the good-parent persona and allowing our inner lover to rise up could have made a difference to our lives earlier. *When* you decide to take that step is up to you, but I do encourage you to remember you are an adult, with needs for companionship, touch, caresses, sex, fun, and all that goes with the territory of dating and falling in love (again).

Sometimes children can hate the idea of you having another partner. It's not easy to handle and can be even harder if you have an unhappy ex with influence over your children's views.

Girls can be prickly about their father's choice of a new woman in his life at any age. From my perspective, girls can be even more territorial than boys and use subtle means of ensuring you know exactly what she's really thinking about your stealing Daddy away from her. If she's particularly close to her mother, then this is even more difficult.

Boys on the other hand might be particularly antsy about the idea of another man telling them what to do, or acting like the boss in their house. It's a basic protection thing for many boys when it comes to their mothers being with any man – and it can lead to problems if not dealt with sensitively, with clear boundaries and open communication.

If your new date's kids have a thing about him dating anyone at all, it won't matter how great a person you are – you'll still be the target of teenage tantrums and can be made to feel very uncomfortable. Teens will smell your fear and home in on it like parasites, tearing at the two of you as you try to create a special new something.

Family issues might be the only thing you ever argue about, but those arguments have the potential to destroy you far more easily than a third (adult) person in the budding-relationship phase.

Dating over the age of 50 is packed with brutal decision making. How you decide to get savvy with regards to the boundaries you set and the ideals you dream about is something you can't predict until testing dilemmas arise and you're right in the middle of them.

Some things you can do to help are:

When a relationship ends, talk with your children as early as possible about the probability that one day you might want to enter into a new marriage or long-term partnership. Naturally, the talk needs to be age appropriate. I became a young widow when my elder child was seven and the other was newborn. Two key things we talked about throughout their young lives were:

1) that I expected they would leave home at a certain age, and

2) that one day Mummy would want to have another relationship.

It was never put to them that this meant a new daddy, but I wanted them to know that I was a woman/adult first, and a mother second. When the time came to have serious or long-term relationships, it was not a hard thing for either of my sons to understand. Their liking my choice of partner was also a consideration but by the time we got to the point of introducing them all to each other, it was at least easier to do based on our prior conversations.

Keep talking with your children but, if the option exists, also talk with your ex about supporting each other in this way. If you are both on the same page about moving forward with other people, then you can both have the sometimes necessary conversations with the kids about acceptance and any difficulties that crop up around the transition.

Rules may have to be set. How will the family feel about your new partner sleeping over? What does this mean? Will you sleep with the doors open or closed? Naked or in sleep-wear? Will the family meet over the breakfast table or does your lover slip home after midnight? It may take a while to get to know each other well enough to even want to introduce your children into the relationship – so, take your time and sort out your attitudes early.

Unless you started having children very late in life, in your 50s and 60s you will hopefully only have older children to deal with at home, if at all. But sensitivities may still exist. At least your children by this time will know what sex is about and that it's a natural part of a healthy relationship. However, that doesn't mean you want to be sitting in the kitchen wearing nothing but smiles as you cook up a post-sex midnight snack as they are coming home from parties or a late work shift.

As a couple, you must both must decide, and *be united in that decision*, about how you are going to manage external relationships from the start. It's pointless to look back later and say: "We should have stood together on that point and not allowed ourselves to be played off against each other by these less mature young adults".

No woman gets an orgasm
from cleaning the kitchen floor.

– Betty Friedman

CHAPTER 9

Do We Grow Out of Slutty Behavior, or Into it?

I was called up by a friend who at 53 was shocked at what happened during a "girls' night out." Two of the group were women she'd not met before. They were in their late 30s. Patty was a lawyer and Janet was a high school assistant principal. Both were intelligent, bright, single and ambitious. They were also single after separating from partners within the past year. The other thing both had in common was that aside from the FM (Fuck Me) stiletto heels and well displayed (but not too much) cleavage in their little black dresses, they were otherwise highly professional women who looked the part.

The night started out at around dinner time but by midnight, only a few scant hours later, both women were wasted. Both were also clearly out to score and my friend observed them regularly straying from the group to hit on men, and fall all over themselves to literally fall all over them. The more the drinks flowed the worse their behavior. Finally, Janet wandered off for the last time and no one was quite sure where she went, despite her "wingmen" doing their level best to look out for her.

Meanwhile Patty called the night a disaster and lined up outside the casino with the rest of the girls' party, aiming to go home for the night with her friends. When their Uber ride was only three minutes away, Patty hooked up with a man who was also waiting outside. She waved off the girls and made it clear she was heading off for the rest of the night with him.

No amount of talk would persuade her that this was a bad idea. It seemed she was hot, horny and desperate for a quick fuck. The others were sure that if it had been even an hour earlier she may have settled for fast sex in the toilets, but no, the evening was done and she was willing to risk everything and head to his place – *alone*!

As we talked it over the next day, my horrified friend and I conceded that perhaps we had a generation-gap issue going on. We were children of the 80s and might have risked a bit for a one-night stand back in our late teens or even our early 20s – though, as already stated, the risks were more about pregnancy back then, not so much STDs. But we didn't travel so much in those days, so were less likely to have a short fling that might expose ourselves to small-town gossip. Maybe, we figured, the women who came after us were behaving quite differently.

The question is: do women in their 50s take such risks to get laid? Probably not, we decided and I've been unable to find a single example of it, despite making a point of seeking such stories for this book. Of course, I'm not so naive to think it doesn't happen, but not quite so readily perhaps. We concluded that at over 45 or 50 we do seem to develop a slightly different level of maturity about sex.

Or do we?

I'd love to know your thoughts.

Everything in the world is about sex. Except sex. Sex is about power.

-Oscar Wilde

CHAPTER 10

The Death of a Delicious Dream

Waking up anxious in the early hours of the morning is similar to the awakening that happens when our relationships fail. Sometimes we know that we were hovering through the night in the grip of sleeplessness that really was never going to end up being fully restful (satisfying) , but we plod on till morning (the end) with our eyes closed, hoping that we' will eventually drop off (get better), even for just an hour or two. But we know we're going to wake up (break up) tired, anyway, because the quality of the sleep was lousy!

When a relationship dies, what we actually grieve for is the loss of what we'd dreamed of. It's our dreams that trip us up, and when we start seeing someone new we're often trying to regain the sense of the dream.

If we get lucky we'll rediscover a new dream, one that is mutually satisfying. If we end up getting 80 per cent of our needs met, we have to ask ourselves if that is enough. As we walk through life as singles, we must get to grips with what compromises we're prepared to make. In later life there are few chances of finding someone without baggage. And yet, we might find someone who measures up for most of the dream we're holding on to. Will you take this person on? Only you can decide.

Those of us who stay married for decades get to know the joy of evolving and growing with our partners. That's not to say it happens easily. Sometimes we have to review what we have, weigh that up against the dreams of what we think our single friends are enjoying, and again, decide on the amount of compromise we are willing to make for ourselves.

That's the key – it's about *us*, ourselves, our own individual selves. No one can possibly know what's right for anyone else, but us. Not even our partners. So, we have to weigh up what we *have* against what we think we *might* be able to have if we compromised more or less in our relationships.

Those choices can be suddenly thrust upon us. This happens when one partner either dies or has one of those not-uncommon rushes of blood to the head and just leaves.

They are out of the marriage and that's that. I met a woman a few months ago who took herself off to the Cook Islands for some time "learning to breathe again" when her husband of more than 30 years suddenly took off.

He went to work one day, and called their daughter the next day to say he was now living in Indonesia with a new girlfriend, and that he was sorry he wouldn't be there for the birth of his daughter's baby, due in a few months.

He said nothing about his wife. There was no message for her aside from the fact that he'd be in touch eventually to arrange sale of their joint assets. Can you imagine?! The wife had no real warning, aside from some *slightly* unusual behavior that made her wonder about his potential to have an affair.

She was just discarded without so much as a single conversation about the state of their marriage. While that may seem like a sudden death – and in many ways it was – for her it was worse than if he'd been struck by a truck on the way to work, because there was no closure. No funeral, no ability to remember the good days and regard him well to the end of her days. He just left!

For someone in her position, trust is even harder to regain than it is for someone whose divorce happens at the end of a long relationship breakdown. But – as for anyone who is suddenly bereft of their partner – a yearning for sex is one thing that is not always a welcome ghost at the end of a marriage or long-term partnership.

Widows who have gone through the anguish of losing their spouse or partner are loath to consider another relationship when it may mean having to revisit such pain. Grief can be a weighty part of the baggage that holds you back from dating again.

Starting over sexually, romantically, is hard work at the best of times when you are 50-plus, but being additionally handicapped by emotional trauma makes it even harder.

And then you find out all the rules have changed since you last ventured into Single Town!

Clinton lied.
A man might forget where
he lives or where he parked the
car, but he never forgets oral
sex, no matter how bad it is.

-Barbara Bush

CHAPTER 11

Condoms, Contraception, and Hair

All women go through it: "My boobs sag, my bum is bigger, my tummy shows the wear and tear of having carried children. It's never gone back to its original shape." Or for the guys: "My balls hang lower, my cock won't stay as hard any more. And I have moobs (man boobs) now".

Signs of aging are evident on my body, just as for every woman my age. I can still wear a bikini and sometimes do, but not so much in public anymore. My boobs are a little worse for wear, and maybe I snore a little nowadays. But so too does the next person you meet. Men and women over 50 everywhere are likely to be challenged by the issue of how we look beneath our clothes. What we wear to bed, our sleeping habits, even our general domestic and physical habits, are all different.

Some people suddenly start dieting, going to the gym,

taking up cycling or line dancing. This can happen in any decade, and frequently does. But the time we reach 50, if we're already well and truly on the treadmill of stop-start body care, we're getting a little tired of it now.

So, do we just give up and say, "Take me as I am, flaws and all?'" No way!

We stress about it, buy new, sexy support underwear, power through the online Victoria's Secret catalogues, and scoff at perfectly proportioned young models who will (we hope and pray) have stretch marks and body anxieties of their own one day.

We buy things we hope will make us look and feel sexier and anticipate that moment of revealing our bodies, hoping like hell the lights are low and that the other person did not ever date a beauty queen. Or if he or she did, that they are perhaps in the early stages of senility-based memory loss. More wine anyone?

The first few dates are the worst. You wonder what the kissing will be like. As in good, better, or worse than you're used to? Does a good kisser necessarily mean a good lover? Ah, no! And great lovers are not all great kissers either.

Then other questions seethe in your head, sometimes while that first kiss is still going on. "When is the right time to take this further? Oh, he's touching my boob. Is that his hand on my bum? Already? Jeez, he's keen. Good thing I'm dressed appropriately – I wonder if he can feel that I'm wearing lace and not much of it. Does he even like underwear? What if I just spent $500 on new lingerie and he doesn't care about that stuff. Oh – tongue – nice, but, eeuw – is he trying to clean my teeth? I miss my ex's whiskers, although clean shaven is nice too."

What exactly are the rules of the game when you're dating at over 50? Should we wait until the third date? The tenth? What are his/her expectations?

While everything is new, the worst part is that it's all affected by whatever we were used in the past. This is where young people have an advantage. They aren't necessarily used to anything yet. And even in your 30s, you have not yet spent more than two decades forming opinions and getting used to what you like.

Then there are the serious issues like condoms, contraception, and hair.

Condoms are still necessary even when not being used for contraceptive purposes. Even in retirement villages and rest homes they are necessary. It might surprise you to know that since 2011, many countries including Australia, UK, and USA, have seen a steady increase of people aged 50-plus contracting STIs including gonorrhoea, syphilis, and chlamydia.

Today's oldies mostly used condoms for birth control when they were young and don't see them so much as a standard part of sexual activity. Young people are now far more at ease with them and often will simply refuse to have sex without condoms.

It is possible to simply visit your doctor for a quick blood test and get a certificate of sexual health – which is well worth having when you're dating at any age. And yes, some doctors will give you a real "certificate" that you can show your potential new partner.

Speaking of health, here's a much bigger issue. What if you're menopausal, but not quite there yet. (It's called the perimenopause phase). Your periods may be hugely irregular, even messier than when you were younger and very unpredictable. Some women have more bleeding "accidents" in later years than during puberty. They can take a lot of getting used to, especially if you are with a new man. And yet on the upside, your new 50-plus man is likely to be far more understanding than his 25-year-old self might have been.

You have to have an important question-and-answer time too. Jack Nicholson asked it of Diane Lane in the movie *Something's Gotta Give*: "Are you on the Pill?" The ideal answer might be a shake of the head, followed by, "Menopause".

Average age for onset of menopause is 52 but it may be several years away for you. As I said at the start of this book, I gotta tell you that asking a drugstore employee who is literally half your age for a morning-after pill is one of those weird moments in life that no one can anticipate.

Might your new partner have invested in a vasectomy? One can only hope. Because the idea of taking the Pill or any other chemically based options when you are in your menopausal years is challenging. After all, it would be pretty darned easy for him to do that, and if he should ever find himself with a supermodel (yeah right!) who wants kids, reversals are relatively easy. For women, the options are considerably less attractive and a lot harder. Most options either involve surgery, hormones or chemicals of some description, and the rhythm method is not reliable.

The biggest challenge with being somewhat menopausal is

that while you know your fertility is very low, you just don't know quite when you might get very unlucky and ovulate. There is a lot of evidence to suggest that a suddenly increase of sexual activity can reverse some of your hormonal resting phases. This makes it even more difficult to read your body well, even if you used to know, almost to the hour, exactly when to avoid or chase that next baby-making opportunity.

Oh, and what about the challenge of hot flashes, which can continue for a decade or more. Cuddling up on a winter's night or in the middle of summer to a woman who suddenly starts emitting hot sweat is not always an attractive thing for a man. And no fun for her, either! Sleeplessness is not exactly conducive to starting or maintaining great new relationships.

And then there's the subject of hair. To lady-scape or not to lady-scape? How much to trim or remove? Most porn sites these days feature bald everything, so men we're dating now are more likely to have developed a visual and sensual preference for smooth skin. Not so long ago, you needed only to ensure your legs, bikini line and underarm hair were sorted.

Men are getting waxed too, now that some women are signaling that they don't like hairy chests, backs, balls, and butts. And we thought lady-scaping was a tough gig!

When we're dating in our later years, all the media noise about hair removal makes it difficult to predict what might or might not appeal to our next lover. And for many of us, deciding when is the right time to first expose ourselves fully naked can be an Everest-sized hurdle. Just as it can be to talk about any sexual preferences, likes, dislikes, and experiences.

I was talking with my beauty therapist over lunch the other

day. I asked her what proportion of her "Brazilian" clients are over 50.

She replied that mostly it was right across the board, from 16 to 75. And why not, she said. After all, it feels better, is cleaner and most of all, the gray issue is easily resolved. And it's not like we are going to line up to have our roots done "down there" right? We may be able to hide our age-advancing color issues at the hair salon, but our pubes are a whole other story. As we age, blond or dark hair tends to go gray everywhere and gray hair is coarser. As a natural redhead (we go gray later and sometimes not at all). I had never considered this – so I leaned in and asked her to share further.

She explained that once people start removing pubic hair, they're not likely to want to go back to having ungroomed minges, beavers, bushes, merkins, or tufts. It feels cleaner, smoother and, quite honestly, the sexual feeling is also improved. It's like drawing back the curtains on the sensitive parts of one's anatomy – regardless of how thinly veiled it may have been. Bare windows still provide a better view, right?

There are apparently marked differences in modesty between young women and older ones. A girl as young as 16 might jump onto the waxing bed without even using a tiny G-String. Disposable paper ones are usually offered as slender cover-ups – not that they cover much but the still do provide a bit of something. Despite having had children and being exposed to many more medical inspections over the years, most older women want to retain a little modesty during the procedure.

I have to say at this point that waxing the hair off your

foo foo is eye-wateringly painful. More than a few f-words are spoken in those rooms. And a good therapist will break out the tweezers and pluck any remaining stubborn hairs individually if necessary.

Much. More. Ouch!

Let's move on to issues around lingerie, G-strings, and panties.

It seems most older women don't much like the discomfort of the G-string, but still love the sexy look and feel of the butterfly or other slightly-more-fabric styles required for date nights and teasing. But under jeans and work clothes we're likely to still go for the comfy Bridget Jones look and feel – or at least something that sits between plain old granny knickers and little lacy numbers.

Gone are the days of "flossing" for the sake of it – perhaps on the off-chance of getting lucky as our lovers drive us home from work ... yeah right! Now we're a little more inclined to opt for comfort first unless we're dressing to thrill. After all, we take a little more time and apply a little more thought to sexual opportunity now. And perhaps because we're more mature, we can tell a man who teases us about plain undies that "there's no point in raising the curtain early for the show if the actress is not yet wearing her best costume".

It also seems that we over-50s are more inclined to want to dress up and role play than our younger counterparts. Perhaps we've matured in terms of our imagination too. While young women love their "cutesie" PJs, most of the sexually active women I've talked with have a special affection for maintaining a serious nightwear collection. Perhaps it's because we know our men are more inclined to appreciate our efforts and to take their time to remove (or not) such items of sleep-wear slowly and sensuously, while younger men are more impatient to reach their destinations.

We're at an age when we want to slow down and enjoy a fine-dining experience rather than just satisfy our hunger – and it takes a few decades to reach this level of maturity.

If her bra matches her panties when you take her clothes off, it wasn't you who decided to have sex.

– Man Mind

CHAPTER 12

Now, Let's Get into the Good Stuff ...

So, you've met someone and you want to start having the best sex of your life. Where to start? With seduction of course.

I met a man who told me that he once spent nearly two hours telling a woman all the things he wanted to do to her if he was alone with her later ... but then never laid a finger on her. They were the proverbial ships passing through each other's lives at the time, and then when they met again, were both happily married. However, she apparently still rates it very highly as being one of the best sexual encounters of her life.

One time when I was on a second date at a very boring movie, a gentleman made love to my left hand – for about an hour. That was all he did – and it was a far more interesting way to sit through a very dull movie than anything else I could have imagined, but it was powerfully sensuous! Neither of us knew how to say *this is an awful film, let's walk out* – but what a fun way to get around it being such a challenging date. Note to self, movies are not a great option for first, second, or third dates.

Of course, the older we get, the more we understand that what happens in the mind is the very best foreplay. But at some point, the Big Moment will arrive.

When, actually, is the best time to "go for it"? Should you just jump in and grab what you can, or take it slowly and be a little sparing with your seductive charms? Only you can answer that, but this question has come up a number of times as I've talk with people about this book. Just when is too soon? What if the sex is amazing but the guy/girl is not, or the reverse? What if the guy/girl is mega-awesome but the sex is terrible? Isn't it best to figure that part out early? I mean, we're all grown-ups by now, right? Surely, we don't have to justify ourselves to anyone else anymore, and we can make our own decisions. But what about the other person's expectations?

The "third date" rule arose sometime in the last few decades – maybe in the 90s. The rule of thumb was that the third date was when you either went for it or went your separate ways. That doesn't mean we have to follow it. It's a *rule of thumb,* for goodness sake, not written in any kind of constitution!

I have been asked several times lately what my purpose is in sharing some deep and personal experiences and viewpoints. Quite simply, I wish to give hope to people in their middle years, or later, that we don't have to shut down just because we reach a certain age. And often, many things can get better.

I've been casually studying sex for nearly 30 years and am a "graduate" of the 80s. As someone who's been single for more years than I've been in serious relationships, I have experienced enough great sex and enough terrible and average sex to feel that I can be objective here.

My current partner, to whom I'm deeply committed, is giving me the best *horizontal relationship* of my life as well as the most satisfying *vertical relationship*. So, it's not just all about sex. That's not to say we do gymnastics in the bedroom – we just take it slow and fully focus on what we each want and need. We also take the time to *talk* about it as we physically explore our own and each other's sexuality.

I should mention here that I seduced him on our second date. This was not because I was totally enraptured by him at the time, but because I had decided at the end of my previous marriage that I was not going to settle for "average" sex for the rest of my life. I had considered this carefully and decided that for me, personally, *good* (or better) sex was a non-negotiable item on my wish list.

I wanted to know up front what was on offer in the bedroom. And so, I went for it – and to my utter delight, it was utterly delightful! I didn't want to go through the elaborate dance of great dating, endearing conversation, and the getting-to-know you phase without first having one of the most important questions answered: could we be sexually compatible?

I have friends who are quite surprised at how I decided to

approach this question. I also know people who have agreed that weeks of slow dates and getting acquainted can peter out anyway, that it can save a lot of time to cut to the chase sooner.

Both men and women have told me that when we get to our middle years, sexual compatibility is usually a totally non-negotiable point. And why shouldn't it be?

A friend named Stacy fell in love a couple of years ago with a man who ticked all her boxes. Despite living in different countries, they were able to meet often for long periods of time and committed to a long-term relationship. They even got engaged. But, last year she called it off. As Stacy explained to me, she just wasn't willing to be frustrated by bad sex and intimacy issues for the rest of her life – and he was unable to or unwilling to make changes in this area.

Why be miserable for years over the quality and quantity of sex you're getting? If you dream of still indulging in quality physical intimacy well into your 80s, then address that desire (pun intended) in your 50s.

Of course, if you're a mentor of younger friends, the notion of jumping into the sack with someone immediately may not feel like a great leadership example. But I believe there is always room for that other great saying – "do as I say, not as I do." (Thanks for that, Pop!) And we never have to reveal our eagerness to anyone but each other, so what do you have to lose by quickly resolving the question of sexual compatibility?

Everyone probably thinks I'm a raving nymphomaniac, that I have an insatiable sexual appetite, when the truth is I'd rather read a book.

– Madonna

CHAPTER 13

Seduction Is Not Just About the Sex

Let's talk now about what you can do to seduce your partner. Whether you're new together or just exploring new ways to make an older relationship work, now is the time to grab your highlighter and make some notes.

Cooking a meal together can be packed with seductive moments. Put on some romantic music, even the kind you might boogie to as you taste food. Stop to dance slowly to an easy jazz rhythm as you slice up the tomatoes. Or try feeding each other chocolate sauce that's intended for drizzling onto the strawberries. It can all be a lot of fun and oh, so sexy.

Let go of inhibitions and try drizzling some of that sauce onto nipples and licking it off, bending over the kitchen counter or ending up on the floor behind the counter – it doesn't matter which! Just commit to enjoying each other as much as the cooking process.

You could agree to set the table wearing only a negligee and stiletto heels. Or be blindfolded ... allow your partner to feed you, kiss you, stimulate you throughout the meal. This is not about getting fed or satisfying actual hunger so much as feeding the desire to spark things up in your sex lives.

A short list of aphrodisiac foods is worth mentioning here:
- Oysters contain amino acids that trigger the production of sex hormones.
- Chilli peppers speed up the heart rate, making you sweat; your body behaves much the same way when aroused.
- Chocolate causes a spike in the pleasure levels of dopamine, although the very *thought* of chocolate actually causes me pleasure too.
- Bananas might be phallus-shaped and so they seem to naturally suggest sex in some minds, but they do contain the enzyme bromelain, which is linked to testosterone production, as well as potassium and vitamin B, which elevate energy.
- Honey contains boron which helps regulate testosterone and estrogen.
- According to sciencedaily.com, watermelon contains lycopene, which may have a Viagra-like effect on the body.
- Figs are referred to in the Bible, linked with the Garden of Eden with references to fertility, but are full of potassium which is good for energy.
- Avocados have been thought of as aphrodisiacs for centuries in South America, but it turns out their claim to fame is

mostly based on their knack of boosting energy by upping vitamin E levels.

According to my limited research, 70 per cent of those still having sex in later life like to indulge in erotic massage. Break out the massage oil and slowly – *really* slowly – explore each other's bodies and erogenous zones. You might be surprised by how much your body has evolved over the years. Nipples that were once unresponsive to stimulation might now be the key to having the best sex ever. So might having your buttocks caressed, or for a man, the tip of the penis (the frenium – just on the underside below the head) caressed and pressed slowly with just the right amount of pressure. Lubricant can work wonders in foreplay. You can get some delicious-tasting varieties now, including options with a soft tingle to heighten the senses even more.

Maybe the feet are ready to awaken to a lover's caress, or the ankles, the back of the knees, inside the elbows, the centre of the back ... just let go and explore. Fully. Slowly. Sensuously.

Try talking to each other about sex ... what you would really like to do and try, and while talking, caress each other's hands only. Convey the feeling you'd like to give each other orally by using your tongue on fingers by candle light ... see where that leads you both.

Sit in the dark and listen to music, curl up with a glass of liqueur each, and some chocolate. Feed each other chocolate and listen to music that inspires you to caress each other slowly and deliberately. Sometimes a "hands off" agreement can leave you desperate for each other's touch. Try it.

Read each other sexy text from porn sites such as literotica. com. See if the senses can be stimulated by sound. Discover and awaken each other's fantasies by reading bedtime stories. Indulge your other senses. Watch a little video porn together. Watch each other put on a show for each other. I think one of the sexiest things you can do is to shave your lover's face after stepping out of the shower, and you know how he's going to feel, taste and then tease you with those soft lips – or stimulate himself slowly while he's looking deeply into your eyes. Some men dream of watching a woman stimulate herself, either with her hands or a vibrator.

You want gold-medal sex? Start with a slow, deliberate attempt to inspire and keep inspiring each other. What *is* gold medal sex? She comes first, he gets the silver medal ... but either of you might then still go for the bronze!

Women always try to
tame themselves as they get
older, but the ones who look
best are often a bit wilder.

-Miacca Prada

CHAPTER 14

The Golden Age of Intimacy

I have heard some say that the 50s decade is the age of true intimacy. It's when we stop clinging to what we think is normal, start letting our guard down and let go of ego. By the time we reach those middle years, we're pretty likely to have experienced all kinds of things, including death – whether of loved ones, parents or friends.

We are maybe parents who have changed our share of diapers and wiped up more than our fair share of vomit – either our own, or our friends' or our kids'. So we know that life is made up of poop, pee, and other stuff that exits our bodies at various times of the day, or month. We may be modest about toilet habits at the start of a relationship but keeping on being shy about emissions is just another hang-up.

I remember a great episode of *Sex and The City* where Carrie Bradshaw's character was talking about doing "number two's" at Mr Big's for the first time. Yup – we girls can be a little shy about poop, but boys are generally not. Men will happily fart, poop and pee and think nothing of it. Women are often a little more reserved about our bodily functions, especially at the start of a new relationship. However, while many of us will let our guard down a little more readily when we're 50-plus, we do want to be clear about our personal boundaries and expectations around bathroom and bedroom etiquette.

Sex is noisy, squishy and slippery, and we need to decide what we physically want, can and can't, or don't, wish to do. We might keep having to stop to find the lubricant and apply it liberally or pause the proceedings to pump up the er ... volume. After all, maintaining hardness (for him) and wetness (for her) over an extended period of lovemaking may not actually be realistic – at any age. Or, we may sweat more, which means the sheets might need to be changed even before we go to sleep after sex. Maybe there'll be a need for little blue pills, or maybe we've finally figured out the key to multiple orgasms – or concluded it's just great to focus on the journey instead of the destination.

At some point, these things need to be talked about.

Our ability to orgasm, or not, the things we like or don't like in bed, our required aids for successful sex, and even our comfort levels around bodily functions – all of it requires us to a bit more open than we may have thought was appropriate or necessary a couple of decades ago.

The menopause stage can mean heavy or surprise periods, or unregulated overheating challenges. Pay attention to contraception if there's any chance at all of an unwanted pregnancy. Preferences for toys, aids, lubricant or libido-enhancing pills, are best shared as soon as possible to avoid later surprises.

My partner asked me before we ever went to bed together to "please not fake it". Thank goodness he did because I'd habitually faked it in the past with some partners, and I was now on notice not to do it with him. His request meant we talked about that and other aspects of sexual pleasure before we even really got into a relationship. It was important for us both to know we could actually talk openly about sex. He had promised himself that he would not compromise on honesty both in and out of bed with his next partner, and I had promised myself not to compromise on the quality of sex.

We agreed that night to commit to a policy of open, honest and clear communication at all times. Sure, there've been some uncomfortable moments, but the results are *total transparency about: Every. Thing!*

You love the idea of spontaneity? It might not happen so easily now we're older. You might need some planning instead – which will also be the case if there are post-surgical or medical issues such as prostate or cancer treatments.

Intimacy is about the love, the care and the conversations you have as a couple. *Total* intimacy comes from feeling free in those open conversations and not holding back about your wants, your desires, your concerns, your feelings. Men and women who have really thought about this – often with the help of counsellors – know that the fastest path to total intimacy is to work on deep communication with your partner.

Trust me, if you can talk openly about how your vagina really works, or how your cock will or won't work sometimes, there's not much else to feel uncomfortable about.

And let's remember that all penises and vaginas are not created equal!

Good sex is like bridge. If you don't have a good partner, you had better have a good hand.

– Mae West

CHAPTER 15

Anticipation is a Powerful Aphrodisiac!

Making love in our minds is pretty intense – and we're likely to be more responsive than ever to mental stimulation. Do you really think that Skype sex, phone sex, or text sex is only for the young? No way. Being able to excite each other over long distances is one of life's most interesting, modern pleasures, regardless of how old we are.

Love letters have been written throughout the ages to tease and titillate; we just have much faster ways of communicating our desires now. Describing what you're doing or long to do, or reminiscing about tastes, textures, feelings or other stimulants can be exhilarating for lovers who are apart for any length of time. If we have the intimacy sorted, then diving into sexy exchanges is great fun – and very satisfying too.

Of course, it does help if you're okay at writing descriptively but if not, there are plenty of pieces of text you can find online and recycle with your own spin on them. Just don't plagiarise by stealing the words of others and pretending they're yours. If you need to borrow ideas, make them your own, okay?

Nothing makes me feel sexier than knowing that at a set time on a certain day or evening, I'm going to be melting into my lover's arms. But when we are apart, the waiting and yearning – both physically and mentally –can be almost overwhelming and so we tease and tantalize from afar.

And then we do what any self-respecting, committed and sexy couple would do – we get creative!

Creativity in the bedroom (although let's not stop there) can take a number of routes with the help of technology. It helps if you are able to articulate your thoughts and fantasies. Writing that you'd like to do certain things to each other's bodies with respective tongues, fingers, and anything else you're both into, can be a powerful way to spice things up. There's also fun to be had in developing your own abbreviations and special language.

Being comfortable with masturbation is obviously a prerequisite – and if you'd prefer your partner to be looking at your own photos, videos, or reading your own erotically charged love stories, then you owe it to yourselves to get creative. Learn to tell a good story slowly and share this level of intimacy openly with each other.

Trust plays a big part in this kind of play, especially if you are recording anything like photos or videos of each other.

And you should agree from the start not to share the material with anyone else.

There is never any guarantee that love will last forever and, should the relationship go sour, neither of you would want your deepest and most personal sexual self to be seen by others. If you both have just as much invested in what you're doing here, there's less likelihood of finding your private moments shared. But do take time to talk about it ahead of time and be committed to total honesty and transparency.

Tips for maximizing your enjoyment of great long-distance sex:

- While it may be tricky if you're in different time zones, pick a mutually suitable time. Treat it like a date, dress for it, close the door, light candles, do whatever helps you relax. This won't be half as much fun if one of you is munching their breakfast cereal or doing chores, while the other is lying in bed and enjoying some deep and meaningful moments alone.

- Decide ahead of time what's good, bad, or icky. Having someone post a photo from afar of a piece of anatomy that the other finds unappealing is a turnoff. Don't spoil the fun by using phrases, images, or suggestions your partner might find distasteful.

- Play a little with the idea of phone sex or "sexting" or using Skype or Facetime first, building up to the real thing. You can't know in advance if it's going to work, and it simply may not.

- If you're not feeling comfortable or confident about any

of this, then talk about it first and unless you are both *completely* at ease, then just don't do it.

If you both really enjoy it, then make this kind of sex part of your ongoing relationship – even if you don't spend time apart. A bit of salt and pepper added to an otherwise dull day at work can mean a lot more fun when you're both free to get together for real.

My research revealed that just over 40 per cent of mid-life lovers are indulging in Skype, text or phone sex, and 12 per cent of respondents said they actively get into it as a way to keep things fresh and interesting, regardless of geographic location.

Just feel free to play.

There's nothing better
than good sex. But bad sex?
A peanut butter and jelly
sandwich is better
than bad sex.

– Billy Joel

CHAPTER 16

Playtime – Getting Down to It

This book would not be complete without a chapter outlining some of the results of the research (as my friends like to call it) into what you can and can't do, and some big ideas for doing it better, longer, or with a little increased passion in the bedroom. Much of this chapter is based on things discovered at one of my favourite stores – Honey Birdette.

Specialist Sensual Boutique stores are the answer to challenges such as:

- My best friend just became single again, and I wanted to drag her off to an adult store for some supplies and education about coping with being single, but she would not get out of the car ..."

- "I really want to spice things up with my partner now that the kids have left home, but the overwhelming range of things in the sex shops means I leave feeling embarrassed and frustrated."

☐ "I love sexy lingerie that fits, and looks hot, but want something truly classy – and don't mind paying for it."

Honey Birdette is one of those sexy, classy adult stores – and there are several brands around the world – posing on the outside as high-end lingerie stores and stocked with only highest quality merchandise. When you first enter all you see is the gorgeous, maybe *slightly* erotic lingerie, some cards and games or gift ideas for brides-to-be. It's only as you venture deeper inside that you discover more erotic styles of lingerie, a wall featuring light bondage gear and another corner dedicated to vibrators, toys, and games.

Imagine you're going out with your honey, and each of you draws a card from the Truth or Dare game pack. One of you has to describe in careful detail your first encounter with an erection – either your own or someone else's. The other one dares you to slip your undies into your partner's pocket before 10pm, keeping it secret from anyone else, of course. Would that put a slightly different edge on the evening?

What about having one of you roll a dice before breakfast, with the other getting to see what the roll's message reveals. It might be "Kiss me passionately, on demand, anywhere or anytime." Or "Shower with me" or, "Let's do 20 minutes (only) of slow touching." If you're too busy then and there, the rule is that before the end of the day, the challenge must be met.

These are just some of the specialty games you can buy,

but you can also create your own versions, such as the very simple, Draw Straws game. Whoever draws the short straw for the weekend has to come up with a really interesting, challenging, romantic, adventurous, erotic or sexy date. You may decide ahead of time just what kind of date it will be, and if there are budgets or other borders to apply. You may also decide one day to sit together and create a list of all the places you want to see or things you'd really like to do together throughout the year, put them into a jar, and at the start of each month take turns at drawing one out – and making that happen.

Get creative!

There are lots of ways to play, and not all have to include just having sex.

Introduce the concept of "touching only" and doing it with love and devotion to exploration. I personally love that this sometimes doesn't even lead to sex but is an expression of love, and a great way to discover new erogenous zones. Waking up to a caressing of the neck, face and ears, is erotic and lovely and sets you both up for great day.

A friend recently introduced his wife to the idea having a pedicure together. She was very unsure, but they went to the mall, sat down, and she was delighted with how good her feet felt afterwards. Back at home, she was then more than happy to indulge his long-held desire to have her caress and massage his feet and ankles.

Erogenous zones are not always located between knees and shoulders. Have you ever had your toes nibbled on? You might be surprised by how delicious it feels. I have friends who swear by this as a form of erotic pleasure. But again, you need to ensure your feet are clean and fragrant. Who wants to put their mouth anywhere near a pair of feet that are stale or sweaty, or with cracked, rough skin?

Speaking of mouths, if you are in (or have recently ended) a relationship that has survived many years, then you may have not have paid much attention to pleasant breath in the mornings – so brush your teeth upon waking if you're hoping for some kissing and cuddling. If you live in a hot climate, just one shower a day may not be ideal. No one wants to start a lovemaking session with body odour as an extra companion. And if you want oral sex, ensure you're clean – properly clean – or you might not get it again, ever.

If your lingerie draw is filled with boring, loose-fitting undies, then go invest in something that works for your partner. Guys also need to know that loose, tighty-whitey underwear is a total turn off for the girls. Freshen up the presentation and packaging just a little and see what happens.

As I outlined a few chapters ago, men seem to be more relaxed in their middle years about taking time to pleasure a woman. This may mean that the man you married 20 years ago who was always too impatient to care if you were wearing lacy under-things – because "why waste good money on sexy lingerie that's only on for a few minutes?" – is now ready for some visual stimulation. Leave some sexy lingerie catalogues "accidentally" lying around. Then, go for it – buy that bra and panties set or the long, lacy robe that is worth wearing with nothing else. And be sure to wash your hair, use the scented soap and indulge in a bit of lady-scaping. You may just awaken a whole new version of the tiger you once knew.

Single men I know of are even more inclined to want to explore the sexy lingerie look, taking time to remove it slowly and indulge in some sensuous touching before, during and after sex. Lovemaking is simply that – making slow, sweet, beautiful love with each other's pleasure, comfort and ultimate enjoyment in mind.

If you still haven't got the message yet, believe me when I say that taking the time to explore what's possible and that inspires you both, will likely lead to the best afterglow and the warmest intimacy you can imagine.

When we reach our 50s, our bodies behave differently than when we were in previous decades. I remember entering my 40s, and thinking – wow, this is great, I feel more in touch with my body physically than ever before.

Most women I know say this happens even more at the fifty-year mark. Whether it's hormonal changes due to menopause or perimenopause, or a more relaxed attitude sexually, or even just that we're better able to take some time to explore our sexuality, there is no doubt about it – the sex just feels better.

Books are finite, sexual
encounters are finite, but the
desire to read and to fuck is infinite.
It surpasses our own deaths, our
fears, our hopes
for peace.

– Robert Bolano

CHAPTER 17

Let's Talk About Toys

Yes, this is that chapter you were hoping for, and may have skipped past some of the others to get to. Let's talk about toys. Vibrators, dildoes, butt plugs, cock rings, whips and paddles, and some light bondage options might also be titillating.

I'm not going to get into anything beyond these main options, for two reasons. One, this is not a handbook about sex and all the ways to use a gazillion toys in the bedroom. Also, I'm personally not experienced with everything out there, neither am I interested in researching too much about the many things I have not listed here. But I will give you some insights into how some of these toys can add spark to your relationship or used for your personal (alone time) pleasure.

Research I did with 50-plus couples before writing this book indicated that nearly 40 per cent liked to use toys as part of their lovemaking, another 27 per cent enjoyed games like role playing and dressing up, and a whopping 70 per cent went for erotic massage. I found 19 per cent were into tantric sex, and 38 per cent liked to watch or read porn together. Nearly half of respondents said they are either satisfied or very satisfied with their sex life, nearly 30 per cent said there was really not much room for improvement. Only 22 per cent indicated they'd like to spice things up a little more.

This is delightful. After all, once the kids have left home and you're discovering your body better after menopause, why not do whatever it takes to enhance the pleasure zones with a bit of fun and some help?

A woman has more than 8,000 nerve endings on her clitoris, and at least one "G-spot" that's often hidden away so far that you need a GPS to help locate it. Myths abound about whether such mystical places even exist and its great fodder for comedians and sit-com script writers.

Science is still arguing about the very existence of G-spots, and it's acknowledged by many that a large per centage (although I could not find actual numbers) of women do not experience any G-spot pleasure, adding to the general mythology that these small, pea-sized pleasure points are not real. Even the *Huffington Post* has published an article denying their very existence.

However, women who are familiar with theirs will relate to what is about to follow. And having discovered mine sometime in the last decade, I can vouch for their reality and would like to share this with you.

The G-spot, named after a gynaecologist named Dr Ernst Gräfenberg, sits about two to three inches (or five centimetres) inside the vagina behind the anterior wall – or in simple terms, the top side. It feels slightly rough, and when a woman is aroused it can grow in size in the same way the clitoris does.

Stroking it gently but firmly – and remember it's called the G-spot, (not the G-area) so direct stimulation is best – can produce an orgasm that is totally different from the feelings you get from clitoral stimulation. A G-spot orgasm can sometimes lead to an ejaculation of fluid through the urethra. It is not urine, having a different taste, texture and smell, but it might feel a little weirdly like it the first time.

Sometimes you just have to expect that your climax will come from a different sensation or feeling, and literally "let go." Opening up to just letting it happen and not focusing on one particular feel-good area, can mean having a totally different full-body or combined sensation of orgasm.

When it comes to multiple orgasms, it becomes a gradual gathering of intensity thing ... the more orgasms you have over a condensed period of time, the more the increased sensations of your body collect together. Sometimes you need to just allow the whole body to simply relax and feel all the sources of pleasure to build. But learning to relax and let go is something you have to practice at doing. Trust me though, the results are well worth it.

Some vibrators are especially designed to have an impact on the G-spot, and will be angled and shaped to enhance the ability to have a G-spot specific orgasm, or G-0.

Of course, the clitoris is also teeming with nerve endings, and vibrators created for C-O purposes supply maximum pleasure there too. Operating at different speeds, they can bring on different C-Os in different ways. A vibrator with a two-pronged head that sits either side of the clitoris will give a totally different feeling from one that sits only on the clitoris.

Guys, you need to know that vibrators do not replace you. Fingers, tongue and penis all create different feelings, and are part of the great pleasure journey. But if you wish to bring in a vibrator to add additional stimulation for your partner – and for yourself – then please don't feel it's threatening your own ability to be the provider of great pleasure. It's just another, different, part of the whole smorgasbord.

It may surprise you to know that vibrators have been around since well before Victorian times. In the early 1800s, doctors would tell tense or unhappy women that they had "hysteria". Many doctors around the world made a good living by offering digital stimulation and relief known as pelvic massage a.k.a masturbation.

One doctor on Harley Street in London, Doctor Joseph Granville, worked so hard at fixing hysterical women that he suffered from repetitive strain injury and found a way to automate the whole exhausting process by inventing an early vibrator. The 2011 romantic comedy movie, Hysteria, told a version of the story.

Back then the female orgasm was a mystery and mastur-bation unmentionable. However, Granville's patients were satisfied, rebooked their appointments, left his surgery with a glow and a jaunty step, and told all their friends.

Doctors for wealthy patients all over the world were soon administering relief that had a remarkable effect on women's troublesome tensions. Granville's invention was a hit immediately with doctors, and then variations were developed for women to use in their homes.

The idea of a machine that could deal adequately with women's "hysteria" was well promoted over the years. Vibrators were marketed alongside toasters and other electrical appliances and used to ease headaches and other aches and pains.

By the 1920s it was becoming clear that personal massagers were being mostly used for only one purpose, and they were soon relegated to the "dark side" of the porn industry. When it became shameful and sinful to own such devices, some women returned to the older option of horseback riding – which was always highly recommended for highly strung young ladies. Then there was "water streaming" – as advocated by the 19th century French – and whatever else they could find and get away with.

It must have been incredibly difficult for single women with unmet desires. Sex outside of marriage carried huge risks. Those who did it anyway had to suffer various consequences – unplanned babies, forced marriages, or worse.

Today, vibrators have made a massive comeback, being almost a must-have device for widows, divorcees and women of all ages from a range of backgrounds. And yes, apparently, even nuns. I know some friends who've tried them and not liked them. One went to great lengths to dispose of hers, "just in case the garbage men happened to see it fall from the bin and knew it was mine." But by and large, many of us see them as an almost necessary item.

Technology is delivering new benefits too. One new model has a remote control. You can slip the vibrator into your panties and give the controller to your partner to play with. During a long drive, a movie, show or dinner – imagine the fun you can both have as he plays with the buttons and you squirm in your seat. Honey Birdette's version, called The Perler, is a lot of fun if you're feeling a bit risqué and want to play anticipation games outside the bedroom.

Many people find battery-operated devices (such as Fleshlights for him, and vibrators or dildos for her) give them much more pleasure, especially if they are single and tend to party alone. Getting relief from sexual frustration is one thing but keeping one's parts in good working order has to be a good idea. As the saying goes, "If you don't use it you might very well lose it." Keeping your options open regarding your ability to perform sexually is something worth considering. At any age!

If you opt for devices you can recharge via a USB, keep them away from prying eyes of hotel cleaning staff and/or teenage children.

Do's and Don'ts:
- Sharing toys is NOT recommended,
- Using toy cleaners instead of household toxic cleaning chemicals is HIGHLY recommended.
- Using quality lubricants that are created especially for the job is HIGHLY recommended.

You can also use coconut or olive oil and KY Jelly is a tried and tested product that has been around for years, but take care using any kind of lubricant as you may be sensitive or intolerant to some brands. Do read the instructions on any packaging.

Cock rings can increase the pleasure for men – and women – in a number of ways. The ring can hold the penis tightly, ensuring a slower build up and stronger erection while also enhancing the sensation of friction against the clitoris. If a man has not been circumcised, it can also help increase sensation of the cock-head by ensuring the foreskin is pulled firmly back.

Then there's bondage. A light whipping with a very soft cat-o-nine-tails, which can also be used to intensify sensation with feather-like tickling is also fun. Being blindfolded and tied up loosely – always with a pre-set safety word to use when you want to stop – can supply heightened sensation and anticipation.

Experiment with what you like and don't like – and ask for advice from store staff when purchasing any sex toys or lubricants. They are generally very helpful and will want your repeat business, so it's in their best interests to share their knowledge with you. They will usually also be far less self-conscious talking openly about sex than you are.

Sex without love is as hollow and ridiculous as love without sex.

– Hunter S. Thompson

CHAPTER 18

You Show Me Yours – First!

As we get older, we notice that some things are just different, sexually. Some techniques work better than others, some things take longer to work, and some things just ... well they are simply different from how we had sex in our youth. Our bodies are evolving and so are our minds.

For instance, your vagina may not be the same in terms of depth, width and tightness. And it's not always a matter of post-birth looseness. I recently heard of a childless woman who decided in her 60s to get a new lover and had to go and get things stretched a bit to ensure adequate mutual comfort. Others seek out minor surgical procedures to tighten up the vagina. You can also now pay for non-surgical tightening, or vaginal rejuvenation, using your own blood.

Leading Cosmedicine™ Doctor, Kirshni Appanna, explained the process to me. First a blood sample (just like a blood test) is taken, then it's spun to separate your red cells and plasma. The plasma, which has a higher concentration of platelets, is injected back into your vaginal wall (the O-spot) and clitoris to help regenerate these areas.

Growth factors in the plasma released stimulate the tissues for up to two years, increasing vaginal secretions and improving orgasms. Developed by Dr Charles Runels, this advanced treatment has become a worldwide phenomenon, and is a relatively quick and simple treatment.

It also works well for men who need extra help with erections. The plasma can be injected into the shaft and glans of the penis. "Ouch!" you may think, but the use of a topical numbing cream makes it almost painless. It's said to be effective in 85 per cent of cases. Some people feel a change almost immediately, but the full effect may take up to five months to kick in.

Other vaginal rejuvenation treatments include a heating device (radio frequency) or a laser that tightens and rejuvenates the vaginal wall, stimulating an increase in collagen and reducing dryness. It takes about 20 minutes, with a local anaesthetic making it relatively pain free.

Many years ago, I heard a gynaecological physiotherapist explain the benefits of using Ben Wa balls. These are two small balls ranging from marble- to egg-sized, connected to each other with ribbon or string, inserted into the vagina and worn for a few minutes or hours at a time to promote natural tightening of the muscles. The weighted balls rest inside you as you move about doing normal everyday things, and you need to use your pelvic floor muscles to ensure they don't just fall out. Some even have gentle bell sounds inside them.

Variations produce increased stimulation and heightened pleasure depending on how you sit and move, and on the weight of the balls. They are highly recommended for women who have had children, especially very large babies, as a means of helping mothers get back into shape and dealing with issues of incontinence and bladder control.

Old Chinese stories tell of jade balls, used by concubines only and kept a secret for many years. They were said to help a woman "milk" a man's penis from inside, barely moving her hips as she brought him to ecstasy while his penis was embedded inside her.

As the easiest way to buy these balls or eggs is from adult stores or sexy-lingerie boutiques, many women think of them mostly as a sex aid. However, they are very valuable as explained above for getting back into shape. You're never too old (or young) to invest in this easy option for ensuring your vaginal physio health.

A woman I met recently told me that in her 70s she was ready once again to engage in a sexual relationship. Her husband of many years had died, but their sex life had dried up nearly 15 years earlier due to his impotence. She had not had penetrative sex in nearly 20 years, and also had not had children. She sought medical assistance to ensure that her vagina was not only well lubricated but was also slightly stretched to allow pleasurable intercourse. A brief course of estrogen cream worked wonders, as did the use of jade eggs to help strengthen and tone her insides.

At 76, she says she is now enjoying the best sex of her life.

Take heart all you 50-somethings reading this – it's *never too late* to indulge in great sex!

While many women might snigger, or even complain about a man's penis being tiny, the size of a woman's vagina is rarely the stuff of jokes and yet the issue is just as important. A very loose vagina can mean in insufficient skin-on-skin stimulation to bring a man to climax. It might feel great, but the journey might take a lot longer than anticipated. Ben Wa or jade balls and surgical or non-surgical procedures can be very necessary tools in getting ready for mid-life or later-life sex.

But as is so often true when we launch into sexual adventures, it helps to have a good sense of humour. Take Nina's story. She and her husband of 20 years had recently agreed to separate but for convenience sake, they decided to attend a New Year's Eve party hosted by old friends.

Nina had decided earlier that day that the New Year would bring the promise of new love, or at least new sex, and it might be worth being prepared. In the afternoon she had tested out her new Ben Wa balls, thought they were pretty easy to use and left them in for a while – several hours in fact. It was only days later that she found out the *suggested* insertion time was 30 minutes twice weekly.

She dressed for her evening out and got a text from her husband. He was on his way to pick her up and would be outside the door in half an hour. Nina went to remove the balls, and disaster struck.

She could not find the string to pull them out.

The string, along with the balls themselves, were somehow lost in her nether regions. Time ticked by. She poked and prodded, bending herself this way and that, but still couldn't find it. Nina was nearly beside herself. The thought of having to ask her estranged husband to take her to the emergency room to extract balls she was using to make her pussy tight enough for sex with a new lover was *mortifying*. To say the least!

She sat once again on the toilet, thanking her guardian angels for helping her to decide against getting long acrylic nails the day before. "OMG, can you imagine if I'd scratched myself!" She pondered the irony and the awfulness of the situation. Would a bath help? No time. Would it be okay to leave them in place? She was definitely growing uncomfortable. Would it be okay to get her best friend to help when she arrived at the party? Oh, now that was going way too far! Nothing for it but to try one last time. Her phone binged again as a new message arrived. "Where the hell are you – I'm waiting!"

She reached inside, probed gently, and prayed – yes, genuinely prayed. Then, success! "I have never felt so relieved in all my life," she said.

And yes, names have been changed of course, and no this did not happen to me.

The older women get, the more beautiful they get. We become ourselves, which is something you can't teach anyone at 18.

– Jennifer Garner

CHAPTER 19

Having to Schedule Sex

I may have mentioned already that at 52 I'm enjoying the best sex of my life. This was a topic for conversation with my hairdresser a couple of weeks after I started writing, and the conversation went something like this.

"So, Dixie, is there much happening for you later today?" That's hairdresser speak for, "Shall I style your hair fabulously well for you or just dry it off a bit?"

"No, I'm just heading to Pilates, then home," I said.

"Pilates, huh. That must be why you're looking so great. You've obviously been going hard at it lately, you are looking fantastic!" Well, if you're having a lot of great sex in a new relationship, you do walk about with a bit of a glow on, right!

I caught her eye as she finished the statement. I blushed, she blushed and we both started laughing at what she'd said. "Oh, not *that* kind of hard at it, huh!" She laughed again. The younger assistant with the fabulous pink hair was looking at us both like we'd lost our minds, clearly not quite in on the joke. After all, millennials really do believe that we're far too old to be having sex after 35, right? At 50-something, we're dinosaurs!

Of course, we chatted on and soon I was saying I was writing a book about sex after 50. This started one of the most interesting sex conversations I've ever had – mostly because it was about the lengths to which some of us will get our share of ecstasy.

For the record, hairdressers are great for research.

We both had stories we'd heard of people in our age group who have to take creative action to have sex.

One example included Jane, who loves sex but has two teenage children living at home, both of whom still walk into their parents' bedroom or bathroom asking questions like, "Mom, did you buy any peanut butter last week?"' or, "Dad, can I borrow the car?" So, Jane and her husband will go into the bathroom, lock the door, turn on some music, and then go into the toilet inside their bathroom (putting yet another door between them and their offspring), so that they can make a bit of noise and really enjoy themselves.

Young adults and older teens these days all think they know everything and yet can't imagine mom and dad having sex, so never think to be mindful of their parents' need for privacy, let alone joyful, uninhibited lovemaking.

Another couple I know both work from home. To get some distance from young adult children who still live with them, they hire a cheap hotel room nearby for a couple of days, once or twice a month. It means they can run off once or twice a day and have as much sex they want without anyone knowing where they are.

Scheduling sex around older offspring is hard work. It's one of the particularly testing issues faced in our hormone-jumbled 50s, because as we get older we often get hornier than ever, need sex more, and yet struggle to find privacy to indulge in some seriously good lovemaking. It's almost worse than when *we* were young and dodging our parents' eagle eyes and ears.

These days, children often grow up and stay home for longer than we did because it's more expensive to rent and we may be supporting them through their university years. That generosity can come at great expense to our libidos.

Our kids might suffer from serious eye strain due to excess eyeball rolling if they knew even half of what their parents do, say, and feel, sexually.

Trying to be quiet in the throes of passion is great fodder for comedians, as are many other aspects of lovemaking in our middle years. We're arguably too old for doing it in the back of the car or under a bridge – but we're too young for denying ourselves our pleasures and too stuck in the pressures of midlife to have enough freedom to fulfil our sexual needs.

Actually, we're not really too old for doing it in places like cars and outdoors; in fact, the blanket on the ground, by the river, ocean or under the stars is a lovely idea. However, it's much less appealing as a *regular* option – especially if we're the ones paying the rent or mortgage and believe we deserve more reliable, dry and private options.

We grab good old-fashioned dirty weekends away when we can, but they get expensive and have to be timed to suit, and so it can happen only occasionally. What are we to do the rest of the time? Which leads to the question – how often do we want to be having sex? Marathons enjoyed while away or while the kids are away is likely not enough if we're keen to have sex several times a week. For some of us this is enough and for others a regular bonk on a Friday night might be okay.

Some people I know are still enjoying quick daily sex, and some are making a smorgasbord meal of it several times a month. We, and our libidos, are all different. In a private study I asked people aged between 50 and 65 (mostly women) about how much sex they were having. The average response was more than twice per week. Overall more than 55 per cent of my respondents were having sex at least six times a month, or more.

Libido pills and other stimulants may be required, and please don't be afraid to talk with your doctor about what's most suitable for you. One friend told me her husband tried blue pills to boost his erections but was put off due to serious headaches and gave up after three times. This effectively brought an end to their sex lives as he didn't want to explore other options. Go figure!

Another (male) friend tried them too, though he really didn't need to, and noticed no difference at all.

The point being – consult with your doctor on what might work for you and, for the sake of your relationship and intimacy, please don't be too quick to give up if something is not working.

Women need a reason to have sex.
Men just need a place.

– Billy Crystal

CHAPTER 20

Spontaneity Derailment

What if there is a lot more to spontaneity than just wanting to be impulsive?

For some reason, I seem to attract random and extraordinary conversations. People often just seem to want to share things with me. How much fun is it to be me sometimes? Lots. Here's an example.

A few years ago, I was speaking at an event that was cancelled at the last minute. All the speakers had already arrived at the international venue, so we did what we could to enjoy this bonus time in our otherwise very busy lives. It was too late for us to rearrange flights so we talked, enjoyed some good food at the expense of the client and had a few laughs in the bar.

The next day, I offered to drive one of the speakers south to visit his family and we got to talk for an hour to two in the car. This man, very happily married, with a gorgeous family, was an inspiration to me. I feel like that about many people who are happy in long-term relationships. By that time, I had been widowed for nearly 10 years, and the ideal of "happy ever after" was still a lovely fantasy. After we'd discussed people and relationships, the conversation moved to sex. I stress again this man was totally in love with his gorgeous wife – this was a purely platonic chat. But we did talk openly about sex – and he shared how he'd had to work at maintaining intimacy after undergoing prostate cancer treatment.

Here's what I learned.

If a man needs surgery to remove the offending prostate completely, he'll struggle later to achieve an adequate erection. Possible fixes involve a pump or injection. Both have their pros and cons but either way, from a wife's perspective, the idea of lying in bed, waiting for your man to either pump up his cock or inject chemicals into it with a sharp needle is pretty confronting to the pleasure senses.

It requires some training as it's a journey of discovery for you both while you find what works and what doesn't. My friend said that he can still orgasm, but there's no ejaculation. And yes, he still gets horny. In fact, his libido is higher than his lovely wife's. For her, being post-menopausal is a more limiting factor than his physical issues. But they made a decision years ago to not let prostate cancer – or menopause for that matter – affect their ability to be a sexually functioning couple. Their intimacy is assured as a result of this decision and their focus remains on making sex a priority in their ongoing relationship.

Imagine a happy ever after with no happy endings!

But that's the whole point of this book. Just because there are limits to what you can actually do does not mean you have to restrict your thinking about objectives or outcomes.

Whether we are single or in a committed relationship, there will be times when we'll hit challenges we need to get our heads around. Spontaneity is an ideal, sure, but that does not mean it's mandatory.

Another side effect of necessary surgery for prostate cancer can be the urinary dribbling that may go on for a very long time. Having to wear an adult diaper can be severely limiting to feeling sexy too.

Another man told me that as a result of a physical condition, regular intercourse was not an option for his wife. He still loved her and had strong physical needs but did not want to be unfaithful to her. They talked it over and she agreed to occasionally help him masturbate. This was enough to get them through for a number of years. While it lacked spontaneity, it at least assisted them to remain intimate.

Some women feel that their man lacks fidelity if he resorts to some necessary jerking off in the privacy of the shower. I'm saddened by this because I know that sexual tension is almost intolerable for some. In those cases, it needs to be treated the same as any other bodily function is ... as a simple necessity. Masturbation is a natural way of life. It's not something to be ashamed of or not talked about, but often is.

It's also clear that some people are low on libido, with almost no sex drive. All I'm saying here is that if you and your lover are mismatched in this department, then it's something that deserves to be talked about openly, and solutions found that suit you both.

The more we talk, the easier our overall relationships are, and the more likely that intimacy can be preserved.

However, I also acknowledge that if you have a brand-new partner and haven't yet encountered problems that might get in the way of spontaneous sex, these conversations can be among the hardest to have. Ever. As we age, we are much more likely to need to have some deep, frank talks. Doing it in the dark, lying beside each other, is often the best way to start. We owe it to ourselves to be willing to learn and keep an open mind about what comes out of such conversations – including what your partner may reveal to you.

Need help to get started on a tough discussion about sex? Try maybe after or before sex. Hold hands, take some deep breaths and speak. You may be super-surprised at what comes out.

No one said this intimacy stuff was easy – but you can do this. And the results of your efforts in this area will prove to be so very worthwhile if it makes all your other communication better too.

Life really does begin at 40. Until then you're just doing research.

– Carl Jung

CHAPTER 21

Slow Sex, Secret Sex, or No Sex at All

More people are willing to enter adult toy stores when we've got some experience behind us and are more open to exploring devices and aids designed for our sexual pleasure.

It seems to be one of the more delightfully naughty times we enjoy as we get older, especially as it's a way of being more open to sharing what we really want. One woman told me the highlight of her 50th birthday was when her husband dragged her into a local adult store and said: "Let's explore what kind of birthday presents you really want."

She said she was more horny then she had been as a young bride.

It's a matter of hormones. At around the age of 50 they can go a bit wild. We're lucky if we are with men who can and want to keep up, and for them it's a great adventure too. Some I met as I began to write this book talked openly about discovering the key to *their* best sex ever.

One man mentioned he was about 45 before he came to understand that maturing sexually was about learning that it really came down to pleasuring his woman. All women. He said that once he figured out that men could slow down, take their time and really understand female needs, sex got better and better for him too, and he was sure that most men he talked to felt the same way.

As a man learns to slow down and explore fully, a woman also learns to take pleasure and enjoy it at a whole different level, and that leads to deeper intimacy for both. In turn, that leads to increased pleasure all round. Because it's really all about connection. The orgasm is just the bonus.

A couple willing to put each other first is a happy couple indeed. And reaching ripe middle age might mean you'll benefit from some reviewing old habits. For instance, over time we can get so used to our lover's touch that what might have once turned us on intensely becomes ho-hum. Think about being tickled. If you know you are about to be tickled under the arms, your brain switches away from finding it ticklish to perceiving it as annoying or maybe even desensitizing. It's the same with having your nipples licked in the same way they've maybe been licked for many years. It might take a change of pace, a new lightness of touch or some fresh sensation to drive us wild. Venturing into a sex shop to find ways to stimulate with toys, lubricants, visual or audio aids can lead to not only sharing secrets about fantasies yet to be explored, but also to totally different experiences in the bedroom.

One couple I know decided to start reading each other

bedtime stories while apart, to stimulate sex via text or phone. Countless couples all over the world are slowly introducing vibrators to their repertoire or have started experimenting with massage and lingerie. Whatever stimulates the senses, works. It's a matter of stepping up to the dance and communicating about what works and what doesn't work. And being honest and open. Again – the more intimate you are able to be, the better the conversations – it's not always the other way around.

I think it's a sad generalisation to consider that women have a lower libido after menopause or to assume we are all collectively slowing down. Now I'm *not* a sex therapist, and cannot answer this for everyone, but surely, we're not *all* hanging up our libidos post menopause? I refuse to believe that – despite the fact that if you search for "sex after 50" on Amazon, you get a ridiculous amount of gag books proposing that it's a myth.

Countless conversations over the years have taught me there are many in middle life who, for a number of reasons, no longer have sex at all and many who are having very average sex. But why? Given all of today's information and openness why are so many of us still not getting what we want?

Youth has no age.

– Pablo Picasso

CHAPTER 22

What Boys and Girls Really Talk About ...

Shows like Sex and the City would have us believe that girls gossip with each other about everything – from how often we can come to the size of a man's penis and how well he uses it. Twenty years after SITC first aired in 1998 today's 50-plus crowd is perhaps the most liberal of all age groups. But that doesn't mean we all regularly dissect our sex lives over brunch.

Women will of course talk about sex. But unless there's an actual issue, most of our chatter is about the superficial aspects of bedroom action. And that's only for those of us still having regular/good sex. Married or single, many of us will talk more about things like menopause than sex. Unless there's someone new or something brand new to explore.

By and large, most people do not discuss sex with their

friends, and that goes for both men and women. When men do talk about sex, it's often very deep and heartfelt because they may be searching hard for answers to personal problems.

They may be no longer performing as well as they used to and want to know if their best buddy has tried the "little blue pill" solution yet. There's been enough joke material and innuendo in sitcoms about Viagra that the reality seems a little daunting for many men.

As one friend put it recently, men go from the "hang the towel off their erection" test, to simply changing the size of the towel before finally accepting that a washcloth might not cut it and *then* it's time to act. Many women will urge their men to sort things out long before then. Men who are single are less inclined to talk about it because the unknown is simply that – unknown. And therefore scary.

Women are more likely to talk about own issues of dryness, tiredness, irregular periods and libido than their men's performance in bed. And here's the interesting thing: while women can talk about deeply intimate things with each other, men will only really discuss their most intimate issues with their partners. This means men can easily end up stuck in ignorance unless they have a partner to share things with. Some would rather step back from a relationship than face talking to a stranger about how things are "not right" for them in the bedroom.

If men are the unusual type who will actually go for regular medical check-ups, then it's an especially good idea at 50-plus. But not many single men will bring up their curiosity about aids like the "little blue pill" – even with a doctor – unless the woman they're having sex with suggests it.

One of my male friends tells me that if men are having trouble getting it up, they won't say anything that might give the game away to their friends. Most will guard their junk and all that goes on "down there" so there can be no doubt about their masculinity.

He also mentioned that men occasionally play golf (or a myriad of other sporting options) as a means of hanging out with each other and indulging in a few wink-wink-nudge-nudge comments. He's noticed during these times how some men reveal they won't give oral sex but will happily take it and complain if they don't get it. Then there are sly suggestions that "Shirley is no longer interested since the children/ menopause arrived", but the men won't take the initiative to make changes. Not even if it's going to save their relationships or their sex life.

How do such attitudes affect the dating scene?

I know one woman who was very put off on the second or third date by the fact that her man had taken Viagra early enough for it to work and assumed they would be having sex, when it was not actually on her agenda. Others have been frustrated by finding that they were ready to go, but their men were not. Getting the timing right can be challenging! Conversations are often the missing ingredient required to help with these issues.

But intimacy doesn't just happen; you have to work on getting good at it.

Some great ways to start tough conversations can include these options:

- ☐ Cook a meal but signal ahead of time that this meal is also going to be about having a discussion about the big issue at hand. The idea is both of you to be ready to talk. It is sometimes necessary to plan ahead to have important conversations.

- ☐ When driving in a car, especially if it's a trip of at least 45 minutes or more, turn off the music and start talking. Ask questions, go gently and focus on what you're saying to each other. Be present. That means not thinking ahead to what you're going to say when the other person has finished but staying fully in the moment and taking all the time needed for each part of the conversation. Practice things like, "So what I hear you saying is ..." Commit to fully hearing out the other. Commit to not arguing – not always a safe or sensible thing to do when driving anyway, right?

- ☐ You must both agree to take anything negative as part of the conversation, treat it with gentleness and care, and receive it that way too. For instance, let's say you learn that your partner has never really liked the way you cook bacon and eggs, but he once politely said they were delicious. Finding out, after a dozen years, that he really dislikes it might make you feel pretty upset, uncomfortable, or even wonder if there are other things he's been holding back on. Just agree to give and receive information with love.

- ☐ Go for a walk. Just as when you're driving, being side by side makes conversation easier. Again – take your time to fully allow the conversation to flow. Don't rush it. Put each other and the important things you're discussing first. Turn off your phones too.

- After some beautiful lovemaking, hold hands in the dark and just start talking. Late at night is best, and again, hold the space open so you can both express yourselves. Listen attentively. Some gentle caressing goes a long way towards softening words too. Commit beforehand to avoid argument and hold that sacred space of your lovemaking area as one you will not taint with talk of work if possible.

I look forward to being older,
when what you look like become
less and less an issue and
what you are is the point.

– Susan Sarandon

CHAPTER 23

The Orgasm Is No Longer the Objective

One of the challenges that men have all their lives is how their penises work. As young men they often had to learn to "unfeel" long enough for their women to get to the point of arousal. Let's face it – girls are usually only just starting to rev their motors when the boys are over the finish line. Race won! Yes! Er, actually no.

A man can get himself off in an estimated one to three minutes when self-pleasuring and so learning to slow down while making love and making it last is at odds with his natural inclination.

By the time he's a man of maturity, the recovery time for repeat performances is much longer, so it's even more necessary to spin out sex for both his own and his partner's pleasure. So how can he do this? There are exercises he can do to learn to control his ejaculation at various stages of his life. If this is an issue that you need to address, please do seek out some help.

For men who can't wait, it might be about learning to "unfeel" and sometimes the distraction of looking around or allowing yourself to go soft for a while is an option. But the older you get, the more this can be challenging too. Having the courage to discuss what you are both feeling is important. But maturity means becoming comfortable with the idea that the orgasm is no longer the objective. That old adage about the journey being more important than the destination is never truer than when it's about sex in our middle and later years.

The point is that women and men do each other a great disservice if they avoid learning about what's possible and seeking help if something's not working well. It's also, I believe, good to understand at least a little of each other's masturbation attitudes and habits.

If you are finally into a mature age and stage you'll be aware by now that we're all different, that you really can't die of embarrassment, that water washes most things off and body fluids exchanged are not as gross as you may have thought when you were 10 years old. I challenge you to come up with one good reason why you should not try your best to get comfortable having some pretty in-depth discussions about sex.

If you are truly uncomfortable, then try the tactic described in the last chapter – take a drive together. Start the conversation by simply asking the other what they may like or dislike about things you do together in bed. For example: "Honey, what do you like most about it when I lick your ...?" Don't settle for an answer that's simply a version of, "It just feels nice". Encourage the other person to actually describe it more. As I've already said, many important conversations are had more easily sitting side by side than across from each other. Try it – you'll be pleasantly surprised.

Start pushing the boundaries just a little – talk about what you do and don't like in a space where you can't distract each other by touching. Be assured, that if your conversation goes well, when you do reach your destination you'll be truly ready to reach for an even more pleasurable one!

Sometimes it's great at bedtime to let go of the need to climax and instead enjoy a meander through the various pleasure points you may both have. While a man may at times not be able to stay hard throughout the entire journey, if you both understand the way you each function, then managing these states becomes easier too.

One option might be to just play for a while, jointly stimulating each other or doing it in turns, reading each other well enough to know exactly where the other person is and, of course, not leaving them on the brink of an orgasm before rolling over and going to sleep.

Next time you turn to each you'll both be ready to pick things up again and this time focus more on achieving overall pleasure for the other person. Again, this is all about communication so you know what your partner wants and needs and understand that what's best for both of you – regardless of whether you get to "arrive together" at the end.

There is no right way to do this. A code that you develop with each other to indicate "this one's for you" or that "now it's your turn" helps with communication in throes of passion.

While orgasms may not be the objective every time, for most of the time they certainly are, and the enjoyment is mutual when both are involved and both care as much as the other about meeting each other's needs.

You know the worst thing
about oral sex? The view.

– Maureen Lipman

It's Not About the Sex!

In writing this book I have been able to expand on some of the "normal" yet extraordinary conversations I've had with people. Some poured out their frustrations – and their stories have made me aware of the elephant-in-the-room fact that men and women plainly most often just don't *get* each other.

While it's clear that boys are different from girls – duh! – there are some things that are very much the same. We all want to be happy, we all want to be understood, and most of us want to be in harmonious partnerships. It's also true, however, that some people are very happy not being a couple or are okay just enjoying each other without living together.

In recent years the media has given women certain notions about the rebalancing of power in the world, but in my view, it has come at the expense of the many good men out there. Women's rights are not what I'm writing about here – I believe in equality, of course – but not when I see the confusion and frustration men feel as they try to figure out who they are and how they fit into this new, more feminist world. Men in their 50s and above seem particularly confused about things like: who pays, should I open the door for her, compliment my female colleague on her new dress? How and when is it appropriate to do this?

Men of all ages don't know what's now acceptable for women who are feeling fully empowered to insist on their rights. Many are even feeling victimized. Today's generation of older guys were raised with mindsets quite different from that of young 21st century men. We women need to be aware of that.

For some men, extremely good manners, in and out of bed, are very important. There are still a lot of old-fashioned values to be enjoyed. And girls: not all men are rapists, paedophiles, dirty bastards, or ignorant pricks – just as not all women are desperately seeking a rich man so they can plunder his wallet.

Why can't we all move past the increasingly common assumptions fuelled by media, Hollywood, and the experiences of embittered people and instead seek to find the good? An example of this is the #metoo movement – which some would argue is doing a lot of good but has also negatively affected many good men too.

Wise women know that a man who is encouraged, empowered, and given the freedom to give and receive love will open up like a flower. This man who is understood and listened to without judgement or fear of being laughed at, will share his dreams, his values, his love, and he will give that love freely. Observing a man who is totally in love, talking about or watching the woman he sees as the most beautiful in the world, is a very special thing.

In researching this book, I was privileged to talk with people who were married, single, newly dating, seeking, straight and gay. The ones who will always stand out for me are the men who were married – men who reflected openly with me on the state of their relationships and how they've evolved over the years. How they themselves have learned, grown, and become who they now are. And how they feel about women in general.

As noted above, not all men are sexist pigs. Not all are thinking only about how to get laid. Some men have been in love with their wives for many years and despite their sex lives being all but non-existent, they have not taken up the options of playing the field, paying for sex, or even making every third shower a long and private one. I know absolutely and without a moment of doubt that there are a lot of very good men, *honorable* men, who would never be unfaithful, regardless of their sexual frustrations.

There seem to be two kinds of people in the world – those of us who believe sex is really important, and everyone else. If you don't really care about sex at all, you're not likely to be reading this book, but maybe you should be. Maybe you need to know there are options, for yourself, and for your partner's needs, to be better met.

Porn isn't the worst thing in the world for grownups who simply want or need some extra stimulation for their self-pleasuring – especially if that's the only sex they're getting. Sex workers also should not be necessarily deemed to be the worst possible solution for a sexless long-term relationship.

When a man or woman pays for non-emotional sex because that feels like their only option – and they still do want to remain faithful to their partner – it's not the same thing as having an affair. Why? Because there is no emotion in the transaction. We perhaps would all do well to understand that.

I know of at least four men whose wives' lives were coming to an end (in each case over several years of serious ill health), and could no longer have sexual intercourse. Each wife made a point of saying to their husbands, "You need it, please go and take care of it with my blessing – though please don't start a relationship with anyone until this is over." Can you imagine loving someone that much? I can.

Say you and your man love to dance, but then you break your leg badly and can't ever dance again. If your partner craves it – and I mean really needs it – would you make him sit out every dance even while the music is playing? Would you object to him tapping his feet to the rhythm while alone and unobserved, or singing along to the songs somewhere if it wasn't affecting you or anyone else in any way?

Why not let ourselves be more gracious, understanding and accepting of each other? We can learn to communicate and share what we want and need. We also don't have to let past relationships dictate how we react now. Turn a new page.

My partner and I were talking late last night in the dark – the best time for such conversations. While we had both agreed at the very start of our relationship to commit to open communication, transparency and loyalty, he wanted to reaffirm our pledge. We also needed, he said, to bring up and address anything that needs to be said on the day, instead of letting anything fester and grow. End of story. Simple really, isn't it.

Sometimes it's easier to decide at the start, and evolve these as we go forward, to have clear rules of engagement. Decide this is how we want to manage our relationship, these are the non-negotiables, and here's the list of things we will embrace fully. We have such an approach to employment, renting property, and education, so why not get all Sheldon-like and have a "relationship agreement". That is not to say it all needs to be written out and signed, but at least talked about.

Committing to these things means we minimize potential for arguments. Issues are mitigated by dealing with them on the spot, not thrown up like vomit during an argument about anything else later. But most of all, it means we can say, "I know and trust we won't reach a point where we allow so many issues to arise that we just decide to end it." This is a very powerful way to work on any relationship and shows total respect to each other.

It's never too late to decide to advance your levels of trust and communication. You can have what you really want ... whether starting out fresh or rejuvenating a long-established union. You can have the best sex, the best times, the best fun and the most love imaginable, by learning to be open, communicating exactly what you want, and loving and accepting each other enough to be totally yourself.

Dixie

When I'm good I'm good,
when I'm bad I'm better.

– Mae West

Sex Trivia – or Did You Know ...

If you need a boost trivia, or want to be 'extra interesting' on a date, then try one of these to ignite a new conversation and see where it goes.

☐ If a female ferret does not have sex for a year, she will die.

☐ Despite her three husbands and a parade of famous lovers (including John F. Kennedy, Frank Sinatra and Joe DiMaggio), it was a psychiatrist that finally helped Marilyn Monroe, the most celebrated sex icon of the 20th century, achieve her first orgasm shortly before her death.

☐ Apparently when Captain Cook visited the Kingdom of Tonga in 1777, King Fatafehi Paulah had been busy fulfilling what he believed to be his "royal duty" of taking

the virginity of every woman in his kingdom. It is estimated that he deflowered 37,800 during his lifetime and
never slept with the same woman twice.

- The sperm of a mouse is longer than the sperm of an elephant.

- Sex past the age of 90 is possible – proving that Age does not matter.

- The average length of a man's penis fully erect is 5.6 inches and size does not matter

- Shaving your pubes makes you more likely to spread STIs or to get one. Pubic hair acts as a gate keeper.

- Women need an average of 20 minutes to climax, men need from 2-10 minutes.

- 1 out of every 10 babies conceived in Europe are created on an Ikea Bed.

- Men can experience multiple orgasms.

- Men having an orgasm two or more times a week are likely to live longer.

- Some research shows that 67% of women will fake orgasms.

- 75% of women cannot climax through intercourse alone.

- A study by the American Socialogist Association found that the most mind-blowing sex comes with being in love with your partner.

- Four popes have died while having sex. 262 have not!

- There is a lot more to the clitoris than meets the eye. It is shaped like a wishbone and is about 3 to 4 1/2 inches long.

- A quarter of penises are slightly bent when erect.

- Nipplegasms exits. They release oxytocin and bring more blood to the genitals.

- An orgasm alone burns 2–3 calories. Foreplay on the other hand can burn 50.

- Humans aren't the only species that partake in oral sex; cheetahs, hyenas, and goats all go down too.

- Male honeybees (Drones) only get to have sex once in their life ... they die after mating because the penis and associated abdominal tissues are ripped from their body after intercourse.

- In 1609, a doctor named Johannes Jacob Wecker reported finding a corpse in Bologna with two penises (a condition called diphallia). Since then, approximately 100 cases of similarly endowed men have been recorded.

- Other than the genitals and the breasts, the inner nose is the only other body part that routinely swells during intercourse – this is because it is made from the same type of erectile tissue as the penis.

- Fellatio and cunnilingus is revered as spiritually fulfilling in Taoist China – Apparently it is considered to have the ability to increase longevity.

- Romans regarded fellatio as far more shameful than anal sex. Not such an issue however if performed by a slave woman. Bad breath was usually considered to be a sign of it, and therefore affected a man's social status.

About Dixie Maria Carlton

Dixie has been igniting and curating conversations with random strangers, since she was a small and precocious toddler in hospital waiting rooms. She has no fear of striking up conversations with people anywhere, anytime, learning new things from people she meets and not being shy to ask tough questions. Her children – now grown – have also become extraordinary communicators and story tellers as a result, and family gatherings around a dinner table can be absolutely hilarious - *storytelling on steroids.*

As a Coach University Graduate in 2003, she's enjoyed 20+ years of honing those skills, and turned to writing books, working with non-fiction authors and professional speakers around the world. Her knowledge of many subjects through this work has led to what she describes as 'a fascinating career path where I get paid to be nosey and learn new things'.

If you want more Horizontal or Vertical Happiness:

Coaching/mentoring/retreats

Coaching options are available on request by contacting Dixie directly. As a certified and experienced life and business coach, she prefers to customise options for direct coaching based on what is needed. Not a sex therapist or psychologist, but wise and very insightful and intuitive with resources to help you move forward in various parts of your life right now.

Other books by Dixie Maria Carlton

Non-fiction:

In the Taboo Conversations Series:

- That **V** Word – *Understanding your values, core values, needs and how they impact on your life every day.* (Due for release August 2023)

In the Authority Author's series

- Start with the Draft – How to plan and write your first draft of a non-fiction book
- From Idea to Authority – Write, Publish and Market a non-fiction book
- Authority Island – Why some authors become authorities and others just write books.

Buying and Selling Old Stuff

Small Business Start-up Essentials

The Power of Promotional Products

Fiction:

Hinerangi – *due for release early 2024.*

The Margaret McKenzie Series
- Song out of time –– Part 1
- Rhythm and Rhyme – Part 2

Hell Hath No Fury

Beyond the Shadows

Please follow Dixie on Amazon for new release updates.

www.amazon.com/stores/Dixie-Maria-Carlton

Social Media:
- Linked In: @dixiecarlton
- Instagram: @dixiethewordwitch
- Facebook: @dixiecarltonauthor
- TikTok: @dixiethewordwitch

www.dixiecarlton.com

To engage Dixie to speak at your next event please visit www.dixiecarlton.com/speaker-topics

Acknowledgements

A lot of very helpful information was gleaned from artful conversations with friends, family, and also a handful of complete strangers as I went from having this book idea to seeing it completed.

Firstly, as I started to write, I was getting calls and suggestions for how to make it better, items to ad and knowledge worth sharing. I learned so much! But first, to Lorraine and Beth at that funky little shoe shop in Queensland – sadly it's no longer there but I still have the shoes! Their stories were endless, and the laughs flowed as did the early inspiration.

To gal pals, and guy pals who opened up and shared their insights and thoughts: Jo Hassan, Karen Tui Boyes, Tony Ryan, Brydon Davidson, Stuart F, Graham H. To Lindsay and Debbie Adams, Lynnette F, Karen W, Julie W, for many hilarious conversations over meals enjoyed; also Beverly for tips on great sex after 70. My hairdresser Fatima Ferizovic-Agovic and beauty therapist Fiona Pram, your insights were exceptional.

This book also would not have been possible were it not for all the people who read advanced copies and participated in surveys.

Special mention goes to Alex and Warren, for endless extraordinary conversations and contributions, inspiration, and ideas. A 35 year age gap between you meant that your combined wisdom was well balanced, and I love that you both believed so much in this project, believed in me and are proud of me for undertaking such an 'interesting' book to write.

And to the extraordinary Lindsey Dawson who editing, and provided outstanding feedback too – thank you. I'm continually humbled and forever grateful to you for being in my lie and your work on this book has been nothing short of brilliant.

Dixie